"Attempts to merge holistic healing and modern high-tech medicine are not new, but the perspective of a Navajo woman surgeon makes this very personal account unique. . . . A voice from another quarter speaks knowingly of modern medicine's discontent with itself."
—*Kirkus Reviews*

"Dr. Alvord weaves a fascinating story."
—*Austin American-Statesman*

"While her insights about the importance of treating a whole person are targeted to her experience of the Navajo culture, they are valuable insights that could help a doctor treating any patient."
—*Albuquerque Journal*

"Movingly details her quest to unify two cultures and two healing traditions."
—*The Dallas Morning News*

The
SCALPEL
and the
SILVER BEAR

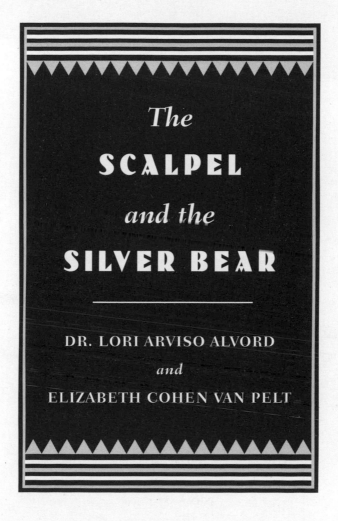

The SCALPEL and the SILVER BEAR

DR. LORI ARVISO ALVORD

and

ELIZABETH COHEN VAN PELT

BANTAM BOOKS

New York Toronto London Sydney Auckland

THE SCALPEL AND THE SILVER BEAR
Bantam hardcover edition published June 1999
Bantam trade paperback edition / June 2000

*Navajo blanket border, courtesy of the National Museum of the American Indian
Smithsonian Institution/slide #22/9191.*

Book Design by Laurie Jewell

ISBN 0-553-37800-7

Published simultaneously in the United States and Canada

Bantam Books are published by Bantam Books, a division of Random House, Inc.
Its trademark, consisting of the words "Bantam Books" and the portrayal of a
rooster, is Registered in U.S. Patent and Trademark Office and in other countries.
Marca Registrada. Bantam Books, 1540 Broadway, New York, New York 10036.

PRINTED IN THE UNITED STATES OF AMERICA

BVG   10   9   8

▲▲▲▲▲

This book is dedicated to my family
and to the members of the Navajo tribe.
May you always "Walk in Beauty."

CONTENTS

▲▲▲▲

ACKNOWLEDGMENTS

A great many people have assisted me in the work that led to the creation of this book. Many were instrumental in helping me realize my dream of becoming a surgeon, and many more have helped me care for Navajo patients. Others were helpful with deepening my knowledge of Navajo traditions, and still others helped me to translate elements of my life and my work onto paper.

My thanks go first to my family, particularly Jon and Kodi, who allowed their lives to be interrupted or put on hold by this time-consuming process across a span of five years, but who supported this project and helped me remember stories of our collective past. My deepest appreciation goes to my mother, Rita Colgan, who lives the principles of "Beauty Way" better than anyone I know. Without your love and protection, I would never have come this far. My heartfelt thanks go the houses of Alvord, Cupp, Colgan, Sakai, Corbett, Arviso, Taylor, Showalter, and Ober-Dennis, for their love, encouragement, and support.

The following acknowledgments are listed in chronological order, as I encountered these individuals or groups in my life:

THE DARTMOUTH YEARS (1975–79): Thanks to the Native Americans at Dartmouth, and to John Kemeny and Michael Dorris for realizing the dream of bringing Native people to

Dartmouth. Thanks to Dartmouth College for the support given to Native students over the past twenty-five years.

THE STANFORD YEARS (1981–91): Thanks to Dr. John Collins and the Stanford Department of General Surgery for their outstanding training program and for their recruitment of women and minorities. Thanks to the Palo Alto Clinic and Menlo Park surgeons for teaching me their technical skills. A special thanks to Dr. Francis Marzoni. Thanks also to the surgeons at the Palo Alto VA, Santa Clara Valley Hospital, the Kaiser Permanente Santa Clara Hospital, and the Kaiser Maunalua Hospital in Hawaii. A heartfelt thank-you to Dr. Scott Wood from a very grateful patient. Thanks to the Stanford American Indian Organization for their support of Native students at Stanford.

THE NEW MEXICO EXPERIENCE (1984–): A very special thank-you to Dr. Ronald Lujan and the staff at Acoma-Canyoncito-Laguna Hospital, and Cibola General Hospital, for helping me believe that Native people could be surgeons, for teaching me how to be a good surgeon and a good person, and for teaching me how to care for the Native people.

THE GALLUP, NEW MEXICO, EXPERIENCE (1991–97): Thanks to the staff of the Gallup Indian Medical Center, and a particular thank-you to the staff of the operating room, recovery room, 2 East, 2 West, 3 West, the ER, and the surgery clinic. Special thanks to Dr. Susan Stuart (and Joe), Dr. Tim Simpson (and Dr. Robyn Molsberry), Dr. Valden Johnson, Roy Smith, Ruby Billy, and Rose Ramone. Thanks to Thomas Hataathlii at Tuba City Medical Center for sharing his knowledge of Navajo ceremonies, and for Kodi's prayer.

THE SECOND DARTMOUTH EXPERIENCE (1997–): A very special thank-you to Gordon Russell for his support of the Native American program at Dartmouth and funding of the

Native Healers Lecture Series at Dartmouth Medical School. Thanks to Dr. Andy Wallace, Adam Keller, Dr. Richard Dow, Dr. John Brooks, and the Student Affairs search committee for their vote of confidence, and thanks to Dartmouth Medical School, Dartmouth Hitchcock Medical Center and Clinic, and Dartmouth College for their very warm welcome!

Thanks go to my co-author, Elizabeth Cohen Van Pelt, our agent Michael Carlisle, and our editor Katie Hall. If believing in something hard enough can make it become real, then you have made that happen with this book.

Finally, I would like to thank my Creator, for giving me life and for showing me that love is the strongest medicine of all.
—LORI ARVISO ALVORD, M.D.
February 1999

I would also like to thank Ernie Bulow for background information on Navajo ceremonies, and Anna Quindlen and David Margolick for their encouragement.
—ELIZABETH COHEN VAN PELT
February 1999

The
SCALPEL
and the
SILVER BEAR

INTRODUCTION

A Navajo weaver takes strands of wool and blends them into something of great beauty and magic; warp and weft combine into a pattern, and the pattern tells a story and has a spirit. This pattern then becomes a piece of the culture and has a life of its own. From the beginning I knew I had to do a similar thing with the strands of my story—to tell how a girl from a small and remote town on an Indian reservation was able to become a surgeon, able to work in the high-tech realm of a surgical operating room, and combine that with another story, about how ancient tribal ways and philosophies can help a floundering medical system find its way back to its original mission: healing.

The first strand of my story shows that anything is possible. The words "Navajo" and "surgeon" are not often seen together. But a minority woman *can* travel across cultural, class, and educational borders and become a part of a medical world whose doors have been closed to minority people for most of its existence. I hope that native people will be encouraged by this story, and that they will follow their own special dreams. The second story is about how I have come to understand, after years of reflection, that my tribe has knowledge about medicine and healing, ways of thinking about health and illness that provide solutions to some of modern medicine's most daunting problems.

It is common knowledge that modern medicine is in crisis. Never before has such an astounding array of medical treatments been available. The latest breakthroughs in research and methodology are stunning achievements and should be acknowledged as such, but along the way we have forgotten some of the things that heal us best—our relationships, how we live our lives, our feelings of wholeness and belonging. For all its technological advances and voyages into previously uncharted waters, modern medicine still has much to learn about healing. Now more than ever, patients themselves feel removed and forgotten, powerless in the face of the institutions that were created to help them. In many ways modern medicine has become a one-way system—from physician to patient. Physicians do the directing, talking at their patients. The other direction, the listening on the part of the physician, is becoming lost. This has left patients without a role in their own treatment. Patients want to be involved in their care and the decisions about how medicine is delivered to them. They want to feel like more than a set of organs and bones, nerves and blood, and participate in the process of restoring their bodies to health. Many patients want deeper, caring relationships with their physicians, and want to be able to choose their own physicians. Physicians complain that they are robbed of the time they need in order to create lasting relationships with their patients. In this new world of "managed care," both patients and physicians suffer, and decisions about health care are often out of the hands of both.

This book is about my journey and my struggles. From my

own mistakes, my own initial misadventures in patient care, I realized that although I was a good surgeon, I was not always a good healer. I went back to the healers of my tribe to learn what a surgical residency could not teach me. From them I have heard a resounding message: Everything in life is connected. Learn to understand the bonds between humans, spirit, and nature. Realize that our illness and our healing alike come from maintaining strong and healthy relationships in every aspect of our lives.

In my culture—the Navajo culture—medicine is performed by a *hataałii,* someone who sees a person not simply as a body, but as a whole being. Body, mind, and spirit are seen as connected to other people, to families, to communities, and even to the planet and universe. All of these relationships need to be in harmony in order to be healthy. Even the relationship between the patient and the healer is important in order to achieve healing. Those types of relationships, so key to us, are not strongly acknowledged in medicine today, yet this is precisely what needs to be given priority. People are looking for a better way to have their health needs addressed. They want a medicine that understands their health needs are not separate from the rest of their lives. A medicine that does not isolate but connects.

Healing is not only a one-to-one relationship, it is multi-dimensional. At the basis of Navajo philosophies of healing is a concept called "Walking in Beauty." It is a way of living a balanced and harmonious life, in touch with all components of one's world. This is a path to better health and healing and life.

If modern medicine is lost—and many believe it is—perhaps it can find its way by looking to the traditions and beliefs of some of America's first inhabitants. It is my hope and vision that groups of people can learn from one another—that the culture of medicine can learn from the culture of Native Americans, and that both can be richer for the experience.

I hope that my words illuminate the importance of this lesson, and encourage doctors and patients everywhere that to walk in beauty is to find the path to a balanced and healthier way of life.

—LORI ARVISO ALVORD
November 1998

Chapter One

▲▲▲▲

CHANTWAYS

Music is a healing force—
all living spirits sing.

—JOANNA SHENANDOAH,
Oneida composer

In many places in the world when a person is ill, a song is sung to heal. For this to be effective, that person must let the song sink into her body, and allow it to penetrate to even the cellular level of her being. In a sense she must breathe it in.

A song, in physical terms, is an action made of breath and sound. It is made by the vibrations of air across a section of membranes in the throat, which are then shaped by the placement of the tongue and mouth. That is a literal description of singing, but of course there is more, much more. A song is also made from the mind, from memory, from imagination, from community, and from the heart. Like all things, a song may be seen in scientific terms or in spiritual terms. Yet neither one alone is sufficient; they need each other to truly represent the reality of the song. Singing comes from that misty place where human physiology, feeling, and spirit collide. It can even be, for some people, a holy act, a religious act, an act with great power.

Today's medical environment provides more healing options than ever for a person who becomes sick. CAT scans and MRIs picture the inside of the human body with astonishing detail; dangerous, invasive surgery has been made commonplace; and intricate operations are now performed with lasers. New drugs with capabilities formerly unimagined are being discovered every day. The Human Genome Project is mapping our DNA from prehistoric times to the present, giving us a better understanding of the evolution of genetic disorders and opening the door to the possibility of someday being able to manipulate the human genetic strand and create "better" human beings.

Yet another type of medicine is also being practiced on our planet. It is one that involves not only the body but the mind and the spirit; it involves not only the person but her family, her community, and her world. It involves song.

The notion of singing a person to wellness and health may sound strange. You may think it unusual of me, a trained physician, even to mention it. But I am not talking about a New Age or alternative treatment. I am speaking of the medicine ways of my tribe, the Navajo, where a singer is called in when someone is sick. As part of the cure, they perform a "sing" or ceremony, called a chantway. The Beauty Way, the Night Chant, the Mountain Way: different kinds of songs cure different kinds of illnesses. A Shooting Way ceremony might be used to cure an illness thought to have been caused by a snake, lightning, or arrows; a Lifeway may cure an illness caused by an accident; an Enemyway heals an illness believed to be caused by the ghosts of a non-Navajo. There even are songs for mental instability.

Not long ago I learned that Navajos are not the only people on earth to recognize the power of the human voice. In places in Africa the people sing to broken bones in order to mend them. Yet the power of a song lies not in a tested, quantifiable, and clinical world and it will not be written about in *The New England Journal of Medicine*. It will not be discussed at meetings of the American Medical Association. Many physicians, good ones, frown at the very mention of it.

Yet one afternoon, at the hospital where I worked as a surgeon in Gallup, New Mexico, singing was going on at the bedside of Charlie Nez. As I stood in a doorway, watching the medicine man leave, I was surprised to see the elderly man, who had stirred little in the preceding days, sit up straighter, and look attentive. I glanced at his chart: his heart rate was steady, and his blood pressure had stabilized. There was a new red flush of circulation in his cheeks.

Charlie Nez was being treated with chemotherapy, radiation, and surgery for an advanced cancer. I know this because I was one of the doctors participating in his treatment. I had performed surgery on his colon to remove a tumor.

But this treatment was not the entirety of the medicine he received. As I stood in the doorway listening to the song of the medicine man who stood beside him, his voice rising and falling in a familiar range of tones, I saw a minor miracle. In Charlie's eyes, for the very first time since I'd met him, was hope.

Any physician will tell you that unless a dying patient has hope and emotional strength, the will to live, a doctor can do little to save him. Watching that hope come back into Charlie Nez's eyes, I realized something else: it would take both medicines to help heal this patient. The only surprising thing about this realization of the two sides of medicine was that it had taken me so long to comprehend this duality, this twoness.

My name is Dr. Lori Arviso Alvord. I am a general surgeon. I am also an enrolled member of my tribe, the *Diné*, or Navajo. I am the first woman in my tribe to learn and practice the discipline of surgery, and it has put me in a rare position of being able to see clearly and distinctly two different styles of medicine—and relate to them both.

In my house in Gallup, New Mexico, the dichotomy is

striking. My beeper lies on the table, my cellular phone is recharging in its cradle, and stack of medical journals stands next to hand-hewn wood-and-leather cradleboard propped against one wall. A menagerie of bear fetishes inhabits the mantelpiece, and through the window I can see the rolling desert peppered with piñon trees beneath the slate-colored sky. I am continually reminded of the simple truth about my life: I live between two worlds. In one of them I am a dispenser of a very technologically advanced Western style of medicine. In the other, people are healed by songs, herbs, sand paintings, and ceremonies held by firelight in the deep of winter.

My father was a full-blooded Navajo, the son of my *shínálí* or grandmother, Grace, and my mother is a *bilagáana*, which in Navajo means a "white person," whose ancestors came from Europe. If you were Navajo, I would introduce myself to you by telling you my clans. My father's mother's clan is *Tsi'naajinii*, the black-streaked wood clan; his father's clan is *Ashįįhi Dineé*, the salt clan. This would tell Navajos not only where I come from but whether we are related because members of the same clan consider each other "brother" and "sister." The clans are the names of our bloodlines. When I introduce myself to you in the white world, I tell you I am a doctor, educated at Stanford University, specializing in general surgery.

In my two worlds I am two different people, defined in different ways—in one by my clan and people, in the other by my education and worldly accomplishments. In one by blood, in the other by paper.

Much of the time and in many circumstances, I am reminded of the metaphor of weaving. My life itself feels like a Navajo rug I am weaving, where the warp is one culture and the weft another. I pull the strings in my life across itself and make it make sense.

My former home embodied these contradictions. It was just one mile from the Gallup Indian Medical Center, where

I was in practice, and about fifty miles from the tiny town of Crownpoint, a cluster of houses and stores braced against the windy backdrop of the high, arid plateaus on the eastern border of the Navajo reservation. Crownpoint is the town where three decades ago I played on the mesas, baby-sat my two little sisters, and whenever I could, read books by authors like Jack London and Robert Louis Stevenson. I read my way through the tiny local library and the vans that came to our community from the Books on Wheels program. I attended Crownpoint Elementary School and Crownpoint High School—reservation schools that are about 95 percent Navajo.

People in Crownpoint lived a hard life. Many families had no running water or electricity. They lived in hogans, or traditional eight-sided dwellings built to face the east, and they herded sheep. Growing up there, I never dreamed that I would someday become a doctor, much less a surgeon. Navajo children didn't dream of such things—we did not allow ourselves to dream that large. We didn't have Navajo doctors, lawyers, or other professionals back then. The Navajo people I knew raised sheep or worked for the government. Some of them worked at convenience stores or for the uranium mines. Doctors, in my experience, were *bilagáanas* and male.

Yet I was encouraged to read and to dream. My mother always seemed to look the other way when I should have been helping more with chores and work, allowing me to disappear into other realms: into the lives of people whose world was so vast compared to Crownpoint.

The fact that my life is split between cultures was one of my earliest realizations. There is a word for this in Navajo—*'ałní*, or person who is half. The Chinese, who some anthropologists believe are the long-ago Asian ancestors of my tribe, have another way of describing it. They called it *yuckso'*, which is also a thin filament between bamboo layers and is considered "neither here nor there."

Even as I type these words, I am going against a basic understanding of my tribe. The *Diné* strongly discourage talking about or drawing attention to themselves. We are taught from the earliest age to be humble, not to brag or speak of our accomplishments. To talk about myself in a book is to go against this part of myself. This brings me discomfort, but I believe that this story is important—to Navajo girls, who may want to know what possibilities are out there for them; to people who wish to think about healing in a broader sense; to doctors who find their professions somehow lacking, and to sick people who may want to look at their illness in a different way. In a time when there is great confusion about how best to treat the human body, to care for it as it ages or becomes sick, my story may shed light on how two cultures can gain knowledge from each other—knowledge about health and wellness, about the bodies and spirits we are given at our birth, and about ways to care for them.

I was born Janette Lorraine Cupp in a military hospital in Tacoma, Washington. To pay for my delivery, my father, who was serving in the Army, poured out a bag of silver dollars onto the hospital administrator's desk. It was about seventeen dollars, and as the coins clinked and glistened onto the desk in a heap, he realized it was all the money he had. Soon, he moved my mother and me back home to the reservation, and I was raised there with my two sisters, Karen and Robyn, who were born not long afterward.

We grew up in the small Navajo community of Crownpoint in a family without money, power, or influence. Most people still spoke Navajo as their first language, and many did not speak English at all. My father was charming, intelligent, and handsome but subject to alcoholic binges, and my mother was blond-haired, blue-eyed, and very attractive. She married my father before she finished high school; he brought her to the reservation to work with him at a trading

post when she was two weeks shy of her sixteenth birthday.
So in a sense she grew up on the reservation as well.

My *shínálí,* or Navajo grandmother, Grace Cupp, told us
many stories—about the people we came from and our clan,
the *Tsi'naajinii.* She told us about the Long Walk, when
Navajo people had been forced to go all the way to southern
New Mexico and were held at an army base there. She told
us to speak English and learn American ways but to also
remember the *Diné* ways. She did that herself, too. Although
she carried a purse like an American woman, watched television, and had developed a taste for hamburgers and Chinese
takeout, in the morning she often went outside at dawn and
looked to the east to greet the morning sun, like a *Diné*
woman. She enjoyed mutton sandwiches and stews, she liked
to collect plants on the mesas to make teas, and she said
she could smell the slightest change in the weather. She
loved to see snow-capped Mount Taylor—the southern
sacred mountain—shimmering in the distance. From her
example we learned that to be Navajo was to be a part of the
Diné nation as well as the larger Native American culture,
proud and strong.

But simply by opening our eyes, we could also see that
to be Navajo meant to be downtrodden and broken, treated
like a lesser human being by white people. As we were growing up, we heard the stories of Indian people captured as
slaves by the Spaniards, we learned the story of the village
Wounded Knee—a place where nearly 400 Lakota men,
women, and children were massacred in the late 1890s by
the Seventh Calvary, and where an armed takeover by Indian
activists occurred on February 27, 1973, to protest a century
of oppression by white society. We watched the occupation
of Alcatraz Island in 1969, where Indians occupied Alcatraz
for nineteen months to "challenge prevailing images of Native Americans as the fading victims of history and a resis-
tance to the policies and treatment of Indian communities

and individuals in the past and . . . the present." We watched
with fascination and a tinge of pride on our living room television set. We learned how the American government took
away Navajo livestock, how they brought in companies to
mine the land they gave us to live on. My sisters and I did not
inherit our spoken language, as English was the primary language in our home, but we did inherit the grief of our people.
It is often referred to as "historical grief"—coming into this
world with the burden of centuries of suffering behind you.
Grief for crimes committed hundreds of years ago that as you
grow older and learn of it, becomes your own. Like black
Americans who must teach their children that their ancestors
arrived in this country as slaves, and the Jews, who must tell
their children of the Holocaust, and like Tibetans, who must
tell their children of the murderous invasion of the Chinese
armies, Navajo children are told of the capture and murder
of their forefathers and mothers, and then they too must
share in the legacy of grief. In addition to dealing with the
stories of the past, each new generation must also deal with
the effects of this grief on the previous generation—poverty,
depression, and alcoholism. It snowballs. As I grew older and
learned more about the history of my tribe, I too grieved—
and became angry.

My mother, a white woman on the reservation, grew to be
loved and accepted by our Navajo friends and neighbors. But
from her we saw what it meant always to be slightly outside a
culture, somewhere on its margin, in a place where we could
not completely belong. We learned what it was like to feel peripheral. This was doubly ironic, because we felt peripheral
to a culture that was itself peripheral to the larger culture
that had engulfed it. We lived on the margin of a margin,
which is dangerously close to nowhere at all.

My parents held no college degrees, but they encouraged
my sisters and me to get an education. In high school I allowed myself to believe that I might someday hold a college
degree. I resisted any larger dreams, for fear they could not

come true. In my high school class of fifty-eight students, only six went on to college.

Years later, after medical school, I returned to work for my own tribe, although I could have had a more lucrative practice elsewhere. I knew that Navajo people mistrusted Western medicine, and that Navajo customs and beliefs, even Navajo ways of interacting with others, often stood in direct opposition to the way I was trained at Stanford to deliver medical care. I wanted to make a difference in the lives of my people, not only by providing surgery to heal them but also by making it easier for them to understand, relate to, and accept Western medicine. By speaking some Navajo with them, by showing respect for their ways, and by being one of them, I could help them. I watched my patients. I listened to them. Slowly I began to develop better ways to heal them, ways that respected their culture and beliefs. I desired to incorporate these traditional beliefs and customs into my practice.

Amazingly enough, as I was gradually allowing my Navajo upbringing to affect my Western medical practice, I found that I myself was changing. I had been trained by a group of physicians who placed much more emphasis on their technical abilities and clinical skills than on their abilities to be caring and sensitive. I had unconsciously adopted many of these attitudes, but while working with the *Diné* I worked to improve my bedside manner, learning little ways to make my patients feel trusting and comfortable with treatments that were completely alien to them.

Navajo patients simply didn't respond well to the brusque and distanced style of Western doctors. To them it is not acceptable to walk into a room, quickly open someone's shirt and listen to their heart with a stethoscope, or stick something in their mouth or ear. Nor is it acceptable to ask probing and personal questions. As I adapted my practice to my culture, my patients relaxed in situations that could otherwise have been highly stressful to them. As they became more comfortable and at ease, something even more remarkable—astonishing, even—happened. When patients were trusting and accepting before surgery, their operations seemed to be more successful. If they were anxious, distrustful, did not understand or resisted treatment, they seemed to have more operative or postoperative complications. Could this be happening? The more I watched, the more I saw it was indeed true. Incorporating Navajo philosophies of balance and symmetry, respect and connectedness into my practice, benefited my patients and allowed everything in my two worlds to make sense.

Navajos believe in *hózhǫ́* or *hózhǫ́ni*—"Walking in Beauty"— a worldview in which everything in life is connected and influences everything else. A stone thrown into a pond can influence the life of a deer in the forest, a human voice and a spoken work can influence events around the world, and all things possess spirit and power. So Navajos make every effort to live in harmony and balance with everyone and everything else. Their belief system sees sickness as a result of things falling out of balance, of losing one's way on the path of beauty. In this belief system, religion and medicine are one and the same.

At a certain point I felt quite sure that my relationships with my Navajo patients were directly influencing the outcome of their surgical operations. Moreover, even what happened while a patient was asleep in the operating room seemed to have a direct impact on the outcome of the surgery. If the case did not go smoothly, if members of the operating team were arguing with one another, if there was any discord, the patient would be directly and negatively affected. Harmony seemed to be key in the OR—and just as in Navajo philosophy, one tiny thing amiss could influence everything else that happened. In response to this realization, I took more time to talk to my patients, to establish a bond of trust with them before surgery. I tried to keep the tone within the OR calm and serene—I worked hard not to allow adverse or negative conditions to arise. I was bringing Navajo philosophy into the OR.

Knowing and treating my patients was a very profound privilege, I realized, and as a surgeon I had license to travel to a country no other person can visit—to the inside of another person's body, a sacred and holy place. To perform surgery is to move in a place where spirits are. It is a place one should not enter, if they cannot enter with *hózhǫ́*.

As I have modified my Western techniques with elements of Navajo culture and philosophy, I have seen the wisdom and truth of Navajo medicine too, and how Navajo patients can benefit from it. In this way I am pulling the strands of my life even closer together. The results have been dazzling— *hózhǫ́ni*. It has been beautiful.

It is my own private medical experiment, although it has not been proven by the "scientific method"—my hope is eventually to help design studies that demonstrate the truth of what my eyes have seen. But I believe it and have seen at firsthand its effectiveness. As I continue to bring *Diné* ways into the OR, I want to teach other students of surgery these things and instill respect for this incredible honor. They do more than fix broken parts of the human body—they bear the responsibility for life itself. In our era of managed care, because of financial constraints and the technological development of better and better equipment, medicine has drifted away from certain basic practices that improve medical outcomes. Emphasis is placed on training doctors to be efficient, cut costs, and be timely, making bedside manner an afterthought. But patients who feel taken care of and understood fare better. We doctors, like medicine men, are in the business of healing, and we must not lose sight of it.

My insights run counter to Western medical practitioners' training. With the pressures of an increasingly overburdened health care system, the tight scheduling, and budget cuts in hospitals, I do not expect it will be easy for them to receive this message. Medicine is moving in quite a different direction altogether. The Navajo view would mean a 180-degree shift for many doctors. But by implementing certain Navajo ways, I believe doctors can achieve better results in their practices.

Living between two worlds and never quite belonging to either, I have leaned from both. A Navajo folk tale tells how some of the stars were born, and I think of it sometimes as I negotiate the thin and delicate line between the medicine I practice and the culture of my patients.

> As Fire Man was descending the ladder from the sky, Coyote stepped up to the blanket he carried and grasping it by two corners swung it into the air so the stone fragments and stardust swept across the sky into a great arc that reached from horizon to horizon. This formed the Milky Way, which the Navajo call Yikáísháhí. It is the pathway for the spirits traveling between heaven and earth; each little star is a footprint.[1]

Navajo healers use song to carry words of the Beauty Way; the songs provide a blueprint for how to live a healthy, harmonious, and balanced life. I would like to create such a pathway between cultures, so that people can walk across and see the wonders on the other side. The scalpel is my tool, as are all the newer technologies of laparoscopy, but my "Silver Bear," my Navajo beliefs and culture—from my *Tsi'-naajinii* and *Ashįįhi Dineé* clans and Navajo heritage—are what guide me.

Modern physicians, who have so much technology at their disposal, must somehow find their way back to healing, their primary task. We should treat our patients the same way we would treat our own relatives. We must find what has been lost as we have become so enraptured with scientific advancements: working with communities, and creating bonds of trust and harmony. We must learn how to sing.

Chapter Two

▲▲▲▲

WALKING THE PATH
BETWEEN WORLDS

*So the People who started from the world
below came up to this White World, and they
have gone in all different directions. They
were made here in the center of the earth as
one people. Now they are known as Indians,
wherever they go.*

—NAVAJO ORIGIN STORY

When I was little, the elder people in my tribe
told me never to put my shoes on the wrong feet—
it was an omen of death. They said not to whis-
tle too loudly, or it might call up the wind. They
told me not to sleep with my head pointing
north—that dead people lay that way. And lastly,
they told me about skinwalkers—human wolves,
people who can assume the shapes of animals and
people and move through the world in these guises.
If a skinwalker comes into your life or follows you,
you could become sick. You could even die. They
told me about these serious dangers in the world. I
did not completely understand them, but I knew I
had to watch out for them. The world was not entirely safe.

When Navajo people become sick, they sometimes wonder which of these rules—and many others like them—might have been broken. If the patient does not heal, people call a *hataałii*, a medicine man, to help them restore their beauty and wellness.

The ways in which we were instructed to live and the wonders of our Navajo world starkly contrasted with the ways we saw ourselves portrayed in the outside world. My two sisters and I would sit on the living room floor watching shoot-'em-up westerns on television, seeing "Indians," who were always the "bad guys," get caught by "good" cowboys and soldiers. The movie Indians were proud and silent, and when they spoke at all, it was in monosyllables. They wore very little clothing, carried bows and arrows, and kept the "scalps" of the enemies they killed. They whooped and hollered, brandished tomahawks, and had red finger-painted across their cheeks. Sometimes they would wander into a Wild West–type of town, get drunk, and stumble around.

Believe it or not, we never imagined that the "Indians" in movies and television shows had anything to do with us. We thought of them as a foreign and bizarre people, like cartoon characters, with peculiar practices. After all, the actors were rarely Native people, so they didn't look like us. And Navajo people are very modest and would never travel around unclothed like that. Most of all, we knew it wasn't right to touch anyone dead, so the idea of carrying around a scalp, an actual piece of a dead person, shocked us. Clearly, those "Indians" were very exotic and strange people. It never entered our minds—until much later—that they were meant to be us.

Worse than the Indian-slaying cowboys or cowboy-slaying Indians was the trauma of the real world and my day-to-day life in Crownpoint. Step by painful step I was learning to negotiate a path between cultures and in the often-cruel country of childhood.

The mesa wind swept across the playground of Crownpoint Elementary School and swirled into tiny funnels. When it hit my bare legs, it tingled like a million tiny needles. It made all the children dance with pain and run for cover. It is one of my first strong memories. It was the early 1960s, and as I stood on the elementary school playground dodging the dust devils, I wondered with whom to play.

To my right were the other Navajo girls. I could hear them laughing and talking in the throaty and complicated sounds of the Navajo language. It reminded me of Navajo songs I loved, the sound of old men singing as they beat the hide-stretched wooden drums. That sound was comforting too, because it reminded me of the old people, but I did not understand it well, and it excluded me from part of the world. My family had not encouraged us to learn Navajo, since it was the old way, while English was said to give opportunity.

To my left were the white children, the sons and daughters of employees of the Bureau of Indian Affairs (BIA), social workers, and reservation doctors. My father worked for the BIA, although he was a Navajo, and my mother worked for the school for many years, as the secretary to the school principal.

Nearby on the playground were my two younger sisters. Karen was athletic, so she fit in anywhere. Her strong body had its own language—it spoke fluent basketball, a language understood by everyone on the reservation. Local and regional school basketball games drew crowds of hundreds. Over the years, as Karen's fluid limbs sank the ball in the net with strength and elegance at all her games, she went on to championships and brought home shiny trophies.

My youngest sister, Robyn, had lighter skin and hair with beautiful auburn tones. She was often invited to play with the white children. It was only I who didn't know where I belonged. I could play games with white girls or run around on the mesas chasing goats with Navajo girls, but didn't feel completely comfortable with either group. I was like Spider Woman, a character in Native American folk tales and stories who wove her life through the world, part here, part there.

I think my *shínálí* (grandmother) Grace understood how I felt. She too was the product of different worlds. One of her grandfathers, Naasht'eźhí, was a medicine man. His name meant Zuni in Navajo, because he lived near the Zuni people, our neighboring tribe. Naasht'eźhí carried a medicine pouch that contained corn pollen, soil from each of the four sacred mountains, and fetishes. These tiny animal-shaped sculptures, made by Zunis, carry the spirits of the animals. The Navajo and Zuni believe they bring good luck and guidance, and act as spiritual guardians. Certain animals are associated with specific clans; for example, the *Tsi'naajinii* clan (one of the clans of our family) are referred to as the "bear people."

My grandmother's other grandfather was Jesus Arviso. A Spaniard, adopted into the tribe as a child after he was captured in a Navajo raid, he became an interpreter between the Spanish, the Americans, and the Navajo. In 1874 he accompanied a Navajo delegation to Washington, D.C., to negotiate land treaties and boundaries. There is a photograph of him with the group—which included the famed Navajo leader Manuelito—at the Smithsonian Institution. He is a handsome Spaniard, standing at the edge of the frame, to the right of a group of older Navajo men, who wear blankets wrapped around their shoulders. The caption describes him as "Jesus Arviso, Navaho captive." Jesús also assisted Washington Mathews, a noted ethnographer who translated many Navajo ceremonies for the first time in the 1880s. They recorded and translated 576 songs from the Night Chant alone. Jesús, along with Chee Dodge (a well-known Navajo leader), translated the chants because they were afraid that the ceremonies would be lost and forgotten over time, and they felt it was important to preserve sacred elements of Navajo culture for future generations.[2] (When I first learned about this, I was astonished and touched that one of my ancestors had cared enough to want to preserve our culture.) My grandmother, as the granddaughter of two men so different in origin and cultural background, also looked at the world with two sets of eyes.

In so many ways I am the product of my heritage—Naasht'eźhí and Jesus Arviso—one a healer, the other a translator. But back then I did not know how to make sense of what felt like a fractured world. How was I to be myself when myself was such a complicated thing?

My *shínálí* had done it, however, and I learned from her. As a child she'd gone from the reservation to the Dutch Christian school in Rehoboth, New Mexico, where they renamed her Grace. "There were five Marys and three Graces," she would remember with a smile. "It was very confusing."

Later she went to the Indian school in Albuquerque, where she said they tried to make her white. To her, Navajo ways were the true ways, the real ways, but white ways were the ones that would help her survive. So she put away her velveteen skirts and jewelry in exchange for cotton and polyester. She cut her long hair, and much later when I was growing up, would go and have her silver-gray hair permed into curls at the JC Penney hairdresser. But in her closet in a shoebox she kept her moccasins, her silver concho belt, and her squash-blossom necklace. Sometimes she would take them out and wear them or run her fingers over their cast silver shapes, remembering.

She grew up in a hogan with a dirt floor where she slept on a lamb fleece. Pet prairie dogs lived in her mother's basket of unspun wool. "If you poured a little bit of soda pop into the palm of your hand," she'd tell me, "they would come out and drink it." Every now and then a rattlesnake would slither in.

By the time Grace Arviso finished high school, she'd become a handsome girl with fiery and lucid eyes. She attended the New Mexico Highlands University, where she studied education. When she came back to the reservation, she married Theron Cupp, an Irishman who helped his mother run the trading post at White Horse Lake. Soon after Cupp's mother's death, he sold the trading post and began his own business: tying fishing flies. My grandmother helped him, and they got many older Navajo women involved in the cottage industry, tying flies all winter in their hogans. It was called Cupp's Flies—

Best in the West. All this time, my grandmother also taught first grade at the White Horse Lake Elementary School. She was one of the first Navajo schoolteachers.

It was while my grandparents lived at White Horse Lake that my father was born. Eventually Grandma Grace became the elementary school's principal.

But my grandmother had secrets. Years later we would learn that it was not Theron Cupp who had fathered my father but another Navajo man—she would not tell us much more. Not until years later, in the early 1990s, would we meet my true grandfather, Dan Showalter, and his family. Our new family members lived in Fort Defiance, Arizona. Not only did they look like us, but our cousins shared many similarities. They, too, had basketball stars in their family, and children who excelled academically.

My *shínálí* Grace's Navajo name was Eihebah, which means "Went into War." Her mother was Biznilbah, or "She Went to War in a Circle," and Grace's stepmother was Nanabah, or "Went Again to War." Traditional Navajo names for women always refer to war (*bah* means "war"). Although I have asked many times, I have never been able to find out exactly why women have war names, when it is the men who go to battle. But if our women did not fight the physical battles, they possessed great mental strength, and they have fought hard for our cultural survival. They have held our families and tribe together. Ours is a matriarchal society, a tribe ruled by women. After marriage young couples go to live near their mother's family. Women are the custodians of the children; in a divorce men cannot claim custody. The lineage of the clans (which are like small tribes within a tribe) is also passed down through women. (As with the "Eve theory," a Navajo person could trace his or her DNA back through the history of the tribe simply by knowing their clans. Since clan members historically were all closely related, a stranger who happens to belong to the same clan will technically have a portion of the same DNA.)

Property is also kept by the women. One's born-into or main clan is one's mother's clan. Because my mother was *bilagáana*, I looked to my father's mother's clan as my born-into clan. I am *Tsi'naajinii*, a black-streaked-wood person, from one of the bear clans. Our clan is also the name of the Navajo eastern sacred mountain, Sisnaaajini, also known as Blanca Peak, near Alamosa, Colorado. The "black-streaked-wood" refers to the ponderosa pine trees that grow there. I have always imagined that our clan and the bears lived first on this mountain. From my grandmother and my tribe, I inherited a strong sense of myself as woman.

Long ago I began to keep little bear fetishes, like those my grandfather had in his medicine pouch. Other members of my family also had bear fetishes. The bear is a powerful, sacred animal to Navajos, who will never kill them. They are represented in many Navajo folk tales and myths, and a live bear was once used in the traditional healing ceremony called the Mountain Chant. For many years I have worn a small silver bear fetish on a chain around my neck.

From the beginning, I have felt the spirit of the bear quite powerfully. The bear fetishes have protected my family. The bear spirit gives me courage and strength.

A traditional story I love tells of a maiden who became a bear. This courageous woman, angry about the death of her husband, decides to take revenge against the canyon or cliff people who killed him.

> *The woman prepared to go against the cliff people. First she took her sewing awls and sharpened them. Then she hid her heart and lungs as Coyote had taught her, and turned herself into a great bear with sharp teeth and claws, and she went against the people of the canyon. When she came among them, they shot at her with their arrows, but they didn't harm her. When she returned home, she turned back into a woman. But every night*

she went out in her bear form and killed the cliff people
with her teeth and claws, but she did not eat them as
Wolf or Bear would have done.[3]

I always remembered that I, too, was of a bear clan and was
therefore strong. When I felt afraid or lost, when I didn't fit
in, I would gather that bear spirit energy within me, and it
would give me a great feeling of strength.

When I was younger, my family went to powwows or
festivals, to Indian dances, and to the New Mexico state fair
every year. And we went to many local basketball games,
where the spirit of Navajo community was strong. Always,
everywhere we went together, I felt the two sides of the
world: one mechanized, rich, and powerful, the other natural, spiritual, and much of the time terribly poor.

For a few years our family ran the town's Laundromat and
dry cleaner. It was a lot of work. Each of us had our own specific tasks having to do with the laundry. Grandma kept the
cash box organized. Karen would unlock the coin boxes and
empty out the change. Even Robyn, who was very young, had
a job—to check the bottoms of the dryers and washers for
loose change and lost items and to clean lint from the dryers.
I helped load and unload the clothes, Mom did all the dry
cleaning, and our father worked hard to keep those machines
working—they broke often and had to be repaired.

Sometimes people came into the laundry from the rez after
weeks of herding, and their clothes carried the smells of
wood fires, the animals they tended, the wind of the mesas.
When we put their clothes in the big silver machines, they
washed out the smell of the wild. In the end we sold the business. It was a relief for all of us to give up on washing the
desert away.

Today Navajo children are still standing on the play-
grounds where I stood, facing the critical decision I would
face after I graduated from high school: to leave the rez, or to

stay and cleave to traditional ways. To let the desert live inside them, or to try to wash it away. They too hear the voice of the wind and the desert, smell the strong smells of our people, and feel the ways we came from. *"Decide,"* the world whispers to them, *"you must choose."*

I chose to leave and get an education, following the path of the books I loved so much. But leaving Dinetah was a frightening prospect. Navajo people believe we are safe within the four sacred mountains that bound the Navajo reservation—Mount Taylor, San Francisco Peak, Blanca Peak, and the La Plata Range. In our creation stories it is the place of our origins, of our emergence to the surface of the earth from other worlds below, the place where Changing Woman and First Man, Coyote, and Twins, and the monsters in our legends roamed. These mountains are central to everything in our lives. To leave this place is to invite imbalance, to break our precious link with the tribe, to leave the Walk of Beauty, and to court danger. It was a dangerous step, that into the unknown, unguarded world.

In our song called the Mountain Chant, each of the sacred mountains is honored. The words describe each mountain and its special qualities.

> *The mountain to the east is Sisna'jin*
> *It is standing out.*
> *The strong White Bead is standing out*
> *A living mountain is standing out . . .*
> *The mountain to the south is Tsoodził*
> *It is standing out.*
> *The strong turquoise is standing out*
> *A living mountain is standing out . . .*
> *The mountain to the west is Dook'o'oosłííd.*
> *It is standing out.*
> *The strong white shell is standing out.*
> *A living mountain is standing out . . .*

The mountain to the north is Dibé Ntsaa.
It is standing out.
The strong jet is standing out.
A living mountain is standing out . . .[4]

If I left, I would leave the enclosed and sacred world within
the strong mountains, standing out.

I made good grades in high school, but I had received a
very marginal education. I had a few good teachers, but
teachers were difficult to recruit to our schools and they
often didn't stay long. Funding was often inadequate. I spent
many hours in classrooms where, I now see, very little was
being taught. Nevertheless my parents always assumed, quite
optimistically, that all their children would go to college. I
don't remember any lectures from my father on the importance of higher education—just that quiet assurance that he
and my mother and Grandmother all believed in us.

My college plans were modest; I assumed I would attend a
nearby state school. But then I happened to meet another
Navajo student who was attending Princeton. I had heard of
Princeton but had no idea where it was. I asked him how
many Indians were there. He replied, "Five." I couldn't even
imagine a place with only five Indians, since our town was 98
percent Indian. Then he mentioned Dartmouth, which had
about fifty Indians on campus, and I felt a little better. *Ivy
League* was a term I had heard, but I had no concept of its
meaning. No one from my high school had ever attended an
Ivy League college.

At my request, my high school counselor gave me the applications for all the Ivy League schools, but I only com-
pleted Dartmouth's because I knew there were fifty Indians
there.

I waited anxiously, and one day the letter came: I was accepted, early decision. I was only sixteen years old. As I was
only half Navajo in blood, I wondered if this meant it would
be only half as dangerous to me to leave Dinetah, the place

between the sacred mountains. Half of me belonged in Dinetah, but the other half of me belonged in that other world
too, I figured. Still, in my heart I was all Navajo, and I instinctively felt afraid of the move. I had seen those who went
away and came back: the Vietnam veterans, broken and lost,
who aimlessly wandered the streets of Gallup, the others
who came back but had forgotten Navajo ways.

My memories of my arrival in Hanover, New Hampshire,
are mostly of the color green. Green cloaked the hillsides,
crawled up the ivied walls, and was reflected in the river
where the Dartmouth crew students sculled. For a girl who
had never been far from Crownpoint, New Mexico, the green
felt incredibly juicy, lush, beautiful, and threatening. Crownpoint had had vast acreage of sky and sand, but aside from
the pastel scrub brush, mesquite, and chamiso, practically
the only growing things there were the tiny stunted pines
called piñon trees. Yet it is beautiful; you can see the edges
and contours of red earth stretching all the way to the box-
shaped faraway cliffs and the horizon. No horizon was in
sight in Hanover, only trees. I felt claustrophobic.

If the physical contrasts were striking, the cultural ones
were even more so. Although I felt lucky to be there, I was in
complete culture shock. I thought people talked too much,
laughed too loud, asked too many personal questions, and
had no respect for privacy. They seemed overly competitive
and put a higher value on material wealth than I was used to.
Navajos placed much more emphasis on a person's relations
to family, clan, tribe, and the other inhabitants of the earth,
both human and nonhuman, than on possessions. Everyone
at home followed unwritten codes for behavior. We were
taught to be humble and not to draw attention to ourselves,
to favor cooperation over competition (so as not to make ourselves "look better" at another's expense or hurt someone's
feelings), to value silence over words, to respect our elders,
and to reserve our opinions until they were asked for.

Understanding the culture of Dartmouth was like taking a

course in itself. I didn't know the meaning of fraternities or the class system (divided into the haves and the have-nots) which were so important there at first. Had the parents of my fellow students taught them survival skills through camping, tracking, and hunting? Did I have any interest in making four-story-high sculptures out of ice for Winter Carnival? Did they respect their elders, their parents? Did I know which fork to use at a formal dinner? What sort of ceremonies did their "tribes" practice? While they pondered such burning questions as the opening day of ski season, I was struggling just to stay warm during the frozen New Hampshire winter and not slip on the ice!

Indian reservations and pueblos could almost be seen as tiny Third World countries, lacking as they did electricity, indoor plumbing, and paved roads. When the Native American students arrived at Dartmouth, one of the first things we were told was that we could attend high tea at Sanborn Hall at four o'clock daily. I walked around the campus in awe, like a peasant visiting the castle of a great king.

The very stately, beautiful, and affluent campus could be intimidating and alienating. The college's unofficial mascot was the "Dartmouth Indian," a tomahawk-wielding red man whose presence was everywhere on the campus, in spite of the Native community's protests. He was like those TV Indians we had watched when we were little and thought so alien. Imagine young Native students seeing white students wearing loincloths and paint on their faces, jumping around with toy tomahawks. Like the rest of the Native community, I was shocked by this caricature.

I remember, distinctly, feeling alienated while walking around Dartmouth's campus that first year. By my sophomore year I understood what it meant to be invisible. People looked right through me—I moved around the campus as unseen as the air. Outside of my freshman roommate, Anne, I never made a close non-Indian friend. I wonder if other students of color felt the same way.

I was very homesick, wishing I didn't have to miss so many familiar events: the Navajo tribal fairs, the Zuni Shalako, the Laguna feast days, the Santa Fe Indian market, the Gallup ceremonial. Everyone at home was having a great time eating wonderful food—roasted corn from the Shiprock market, posole, red chile stew, venison jerky—and I was stuck in a library far away. I missed watching the Apache Devil Dancers and the Pueblo Buffalo Dancers. I missed the sight of Navajo traditional clothing, emblazoned with silver and turquoise, and the pink-and-purple-splashed sunsets of New Mexico. I missed that smell—that small we had tried to wash away at our laundromat so long ago—the smell of wildness, the desert, and the Navajo world.

Sometimes I wondered: If I'd had a *kinaałdá* ceremony, could I have been stronger, more independent, better able to face this loneliness and alienation, less unassured. The *kinaałdá* is part of the Blessing Way set of ceremonies performed for girls when they reach puberty. Blessing Way tells the story of Changing Woman (a central Navajo diety), and the *kinaałdá* celebrates her coming into womanhood. The family and community gather around her, she is sung to, and her female relatives massage her from head to toe, giving her the power and strength of womanhood. A large corn cake is baked underground in a corn husk–lined pit, and the girl sprinkles cornmeal over the top. Each day for four days, she runs for a mile toward the new sun, toward her new life. It gives a young woman strength and power, confidence and se-curity, as she goes through menses for the first time. She takes that strength and those "good thoughts" with her into the world. I could have used that assurance. Because my family was less traditional, my sisters and I did not have *kinaałdá* ceremonies, although we attended those of our cousins. Nevertheless, since the Navajo culture is matri-archal, I think I was better prepared as a woman in a "man's world" than many white women I met.

A few things at Dartmouth, however, were comforting and

did make me feel at home. For one thing, dogs roamed the campus freely. They didn't belong to anybody in particular but to everybody and were fed and cared for by the entire campus. Muttlike, wily, always after something to eat, they reminded me naturally of rez dogs. And everywhere I looked playful squirrels ran around, reminding me of the prairie dogs who run around their prairie dog cities on the mesas and sit up on their hind legs to watch the cars drive by.

Academically, due to my strong reading background, I held my own in classes like literature and social sciences, but I was completely unprepared for the physical and life sciences. After receiving the only D of my entire life in calculus, I retreated from the sciences altogether. The high school at Crownpoint had not prepared me adequately to compete with the Ivy Leaguers. Futhermore, I had an additional problem. As I mentioned earlier, Navajos are taught from the youngest age never to draw attention to ourselves. So Navajo children do not raise their hands in class. At a school like Dartmouth, the lack of participation was seen as a sign not of humility but lack of interest and a disengaged attitude. My Navajo humility was combined with a deep feeling of academic inferiority; it was hard to compete with students who had taken calculus and read Chaucer in high school. I sat in the back and tried not to reveal my ignorance.

This sense of being torn between worlds was reflected even in my studies: I chose a double major, psychology and sociology, modified with Native American studies. I received honors in my freshman seminar as well as in two Native American studies courses that stressed writing. As a result, I found myself thinking of teaching Native American studies as a career, and perhaps also becoming a writer.

In fact, I loved Dartmouth's Native American program. It had the tough job of recruiting students like us, who were very high risk. We frequently had had only marginal high school preparation; many were reluctant to come to school so far from home; and like skittish wild horses, some would turn tail and run home at the least provocation. We found great comfort in one another, for although we came from many different tribes, our experiences at Dartmouth were similar: We all felt disconnected from the mainstream student body. For the women, it was even worse. At the time I arrived on the scene, Dartmouth had only recently changed from an all-male to a coed student body, and many of the men resented the presence of women on campus. Referred to as cohogs instead of coeds, women were shunned for dates; instead girls were bused in from nearby women's colleges on weekends. Social life was dominated by the fraternities, and, if we went to their parties at all, we were often ignored.

For all these reasons, the few Native American students at Dartmouth coalesced into a solid community who did almost everything together. Our group was made up of Paiutes, Sioux, Cherokees, Chippewas, Navajos, Pueblos, and many other tribes. We were friends, lovers, rivals, enemies. I have been a part of many other groups since then, but nothing compared in intensity to the experience of being a member of that Native American student group.

Though we often felt as though we didn't belong at Dartmouth, the ironic truth is that we did belong, or rather, we were entitled to be there. Eleazar Wheelock, the Connecticut minister who founded Dartmouth College in 1769, did so with funds that came from King George III, who wished to establish a place to "educate the savages." The college flourished, but for literally hundreds of years its original founding purpose was not honored. "Educating savages" was not on the real agenda; it had simply been a way to get land and money. Before the 1960s fewer than twenty Native students graduated from Dartmouth. Then in the 1970s the Native American studies program was developed by college president John Kemeny and writer Michael Dorris, and Dartmouth began to take its mission in earnest.

We all knew the primary reason why we were there.

Without the vision of Kemeny and Dorris, we would never have had an opportunity to set foot on the grounds of such an institution, let alone actually enroll. We were there because of the generous scholarships the college had given us, and the money from our tribes.

Some years later, reflecting back on my college experiences, I realized something else. Much of the outside, non-Indian world is tribeless, full of wandering singular souls, seeking connection through societies, clubs, and other groups. White people know what it is to be a family, but to be a tribe is something of an altogether different sort. It provides a feeling of inclusion in something larger, of having a set place in the universe where one always belongs. It provides connectedness and a blueprint for how to live.

At Dartmouth the fraternities and sororities seemed to be attempts to claim or create tribes. Their activities often seemed to me to be unconscious re-creations of rituals and initiation ceremonies. But the fraternities emphasized exclusion as much as inclusion, and their rituals involved alcohol and hazing initiations. Although they developed from a natural urge for community, they lacked much that a real tribe has.

I began to honor and cherish my tribal membership, and in the years that followed I came to understand that such membership is central to mental health, to spiritual health, to physical health. A tribe is a community of people connected by blood or heart, by geography and tradition, who help one another and share a belief system. Community and tribe not only reduce the alienation people feel but in doing so stave off illness. In a sense they are a form of preventive medicine. Most Americans have lost their tribal identities, although at one time, most likely, everyone belonged to a tribe. One way to remedy this is to find and establish groups of people who can nurture and support one another. The Native American students at Dartmouth had become such a group.

Our new "tribe" had its ceremonies. Each year, in a primitive outdoor amphitheater called the Bema where concerts and plays were sometimes put on, we held a campus pow-wow. Feathered fancy dancers and women in "jingle dresses" or in beaded and brightly colored fabric would spin and step to the drums of Plains Indians or to songs from an invited singer from a pueblo. The women would whirl, their shawls swirling and twisting into corkscrew shapes around them. They'd dance to two big hide-stretched drums, encircled by the men, who struck the drums rhythmically and sang. Their voices wove and resonated, rose and fell above the steady heartbeat of the drums. This ceremony was a chance for the Native and non-Native communities to come together as one. I felt then, briefly, that I belonged.

In the evening after the powwow the singing and drumming would continue at a party called a "49"—but here the ancient rhythms were mixed with modern English lyrics. The songs we sang could be romantic, funny, or political; they could be about reservation life and pickup trucks or the Bureau of Indian Affairs. They always sounded the same though, with a blend of voices rising around a drumbeat, and a melody that pulled out our memories of childhood songs.

Dartmouth was good for me. Singing with the other students melted some of my historical grief and anger into a larger powerful force, a force I would take with me into the world. I gained a new kind of family and tribe, with new songs that held us together. Once again, songs had the power to heal.

Chapter Three

▲▲▲▲

JOURNEY DOWN
THE MEDICINE PATH

In high school I had been fascinated by the human body—the various systems inside it seemed to me like the earth in miniature. Like the tides and currents of the oceans, it had the rivers and capillary tributaries of blood. Instead of an atmosphere, it had the processes of breathing and oxygenation. Bone and sinew underlay it all, like the rocks inside the earth. And it offered mysteries as well: how did all these systems work together to make a whole human being?

When I was about fourteen, I worked for a while at a reservation pharmacy in Crownpoint. I was much impressed by the amount of information the pharmacists seemed to hold in their heads about medications and bodies. The names of the medicines seemed so complicated and long with multiple names for each one—a generic and sometimes several brand names. How did each of them work? And the pharmacists knew so much peripheral information as well—which drug would have what side effects on whom, which drug would or would not go with another drug. What part of the body did each drug affect? And above all, how could any one person learn so much?

In the school library I paged through the "human body" section of the encyclopedia, staring at the translucent pages that represented the different systems—lymphatic, skeletal, muscular. When all the pages were laid together they made a complete human body. Where in this scheme, I wondered, did the human soul reside? Maybe the soul was the clear, delicate plastic pages themselves—invisible, magic, and transparent.

When I finished Dartmouth in 1979, I thought of those transparent pages. I wished I could peel away the layers of myself and find the deepest thing inside me. If I just looked deep enough, I thought, I could find the truth, like a white, undeniable bone structure.

On a visit home I realized that finding work on the rez would be next to impossible, so I looked for a job in Albuquerque, the nearest reasonable-sized city. It was during the recession of the early 1980s, and there wasn't much out there in the way of entry-level positions. Every day, with a ballpoint pen and a notepad, I scoured the *Albuquerque Journal*'s classifieds, circling possibilities and jotting down phone numbers. One morning I saw an ad for a social worker for Bernalillo County—something I might be borderline eligible for with my social sciences background. I applied for the job and was offered the position. But at the last minute, just before accepting it, I found out about another opening. A position was available for a research assistant on brain physiology, working for a medical researcher named Dr. Gary Rosenberg, at the University of New Mexico. It seemed exciting, different, and interesting. After a brief talk with Dr. Rosenberg, he offered me the position, and I accepted.

There was absolutely nothing practical about the job. The pay was abysmal—a barely livable $9,000 a year, $4,000 less than the social worker position. And it turned out to be considerably less glamorous than it appeared.

I prepared Dr. Rosenberg's chemical solutions to store tissue samples, and I carefully weighed and labeled specimens. I cleaned up the lab. I had interesting discussions with him about his research.

One day as I was working, he stopped me. "Lori, have you ever thought about going to medical school?" I'm sure I visibly balked. A Navajo woman physician. I couldn't remember ever hearing of one in my entire life. "No, really, I'm serious," he said. "Maybe you *should* think about it."

I blushed as I dropped my eyes and turned back to my work. I vividly recalled my dismal brush with the physical and life sciences at Dartmouth. *I don't have what it takes,* I thought.

Yet as soon he spoke the words, I began to take the idea seriously. In traditional Navajo belief, speaking a thought into the air gives it more power.

My new fascination with brain research, the magic pills in the pharmacy, and the mysterious plastic pages in the encyclopedia all joined together to begin to defy my science fears from Dartmouth. I'd walked into Dr. Rosenberg's lab cold, with no research experience, but I somehow found the concepts and mechanics of his experiments easy to grasp. Soon I was spending less time cleaning laboratory counters and more time running data through computer statistical packages, like the ones that I'd worked with in psychology classes.

After a few weeks of thinking about his question I made up my mind: I would try the sciences again—just as an experiment—in a few premed classes at the University of New Mexico. With a generous amount of anxiety (I felt as if I were creeping up on a large sleeping bear), I enrolled in a night course on biology, which seemed the easiest science to "overtake."

To my relief, I did well. In biology class, I was enchanted by the mechanics of human physiology: that a single cell, with its process of mitosis, could become an entire organism; that a chain of DNA, like a spiral staircase, could hold the secret recipe for an entire organism; that an organism could survive illness and disease through its immune system, which would "fight back." Stunning. Again, the system seemed to have the ability to attain balance, like the planet. The body was very much like the Navajo philosophy of the universe. It had *hózhó*. It was beautiful.

I decided to go a step further and take on one of the real monsters. So, while still working full-time, I went to a physics class on my lunch breaks. I thought, if I can handle this, then I will take all the premed classes and apply to medical school.

A few weeks later I went back to Dr. Rosenberg. "I want to quit my job."

"Why?" he asked. "Is something wrong?" I told him that, to my surprise, I was doing well in physics.

My interest in this scientific way of looking at the world was magnified with each class I took. Biochemistry, chemistry, anatomy, physiology, even calculus had the same internal logic as much Native American cosmology. The way the white blood cells attack an intruding virus, the way too much or too little of anything disturbs the body functions, the way tissue defends or repairs itself—it was all *hózhó*, the beautiful balance of the universe, rephrased in scientific terms.

Seeing the connections between the two cosmologies, Navajo and scientific, I felt a new passion begin to grow inside me.

"I want to go back to school—full-time—and apply to med school," I said to Rosenberg. His reaction was very subtle—a suggestion of a smile flickered over his face. "I think that's a good decision, Lori," he said.

No funding was available to help finance my premed classes, and it was rough financially for a while. A lot of dinners consisted of beans and rice. I didn't talk to people about my plans because I didn't want to have to do any explaining if I wasn't accepted into medical school. My family was fairly neutral—they gave me no words of discouragement, but no cheerleading either. I think, like most parents, they were worried I'd be hurt if the dream didn't come true. One afternoon, over a stern-looking steel desk in a sparse office at the university, an adviser told me not to get my hopes up. But in spite of his words I was hopeful, I took the MCATs (Medical College Admission exams) and applied to several of the very best schools in the country (my dream schools) and then to a few others, including the University of New Mexico (my reality schools).

A few months later I received the news: I'd been accepted at two top medical schools—UC San Francisco and Stanford. After what the UNM adviser had told me I was very surprised. Many factors must have contributed to my acceptance at these top schools, among them most certainly my graduation from Dartmouth and my being a Native American woman. In the early 1980s admitting a percentage of minorities was still considered a good, fair, and balanced aim; it was not disparaged as meeting a "quota." I like to think that I won the award for "the longest distance traveled."

I'd applied to the Bay Area schools not only because they were some of the best, but also because my sister Karen was at Stanford, and I wanted to live near her. My father, who had once wanted to go to medical school himself, was very excited (now that it was safe for him to be so!). I visited both UC San Francisco and Stanford and fell in love with Stanford's stately colonial Hispanic arches, red-tile-roofed buildings, and gracious, long-limbed, ancient eucalyptus trees, which cast shade over the campus and tunneled the avenues.

I was also drawn by Stanford's large and active Native American community, which had its own cozy building with pictures of its members, with their names and their tribes written below. I knew from Karen that they could be very supportive when or if things got difficult. In the end, even though San Francisco was rated the best medical school in the country at the time, I chose Stanford.

My father went all around the rez in his pickup truck telling everyone that his two daughters were going to Stanford and one was in medical school. He had not known what to make of Dartmouth, distant and eastern, but California and Stanford were in his vernacular. They were West. Soon he helped me pack up, and we drove to Palo Alto, where I moved to a neighborhood close to Karen.

In spite of having my sister near, my first years at Stanford were difficult. Once again I was an outsider—outside the sacred mountains—and it was often lonely and unsettling. I spent my evenings and weekends studying in the Fleischman Learning Center, usually alone. My class of eighty-six students included only two other Native Americans: Robert Fairbanks, a Chippewa from Minnesota, and Migue Dozier, from Santa Clara Pueblo in New Mexico. The very thought of exhibiting my skills and knowledge before others was disturbing: I could not bring myself to participate in class discussions and debates, or to volunteer answers to professors' questions, although it was expected. The same problems I had encountered at Dartmouth were even more exaggerated here. I didn't feel comfortable raising my hand in class, I wasn't competitive enough about test scores and projects, and I didn't like to draw attention to myself. I lacked the "right stuff" that every med student needs: a competitive edge. Yet it was hard for me to behave any other way. Silence is a normal part of Navajo communication; words are used sparingly and weighed carefully. It took me a long time to be comfortable with the non-Navajo style of learning.

Still, I found once again what I had always been attracted to: the natural logic of the human body, its systems of balance and order that make sense much as Navajo philosophy makes sense. As I memorized the name of every bone and tendon and blood vessel they seemed like the names of animals or trees. There is great power in knowing the name of something.

▲▲▲▲

Soon after I started my medical studies, I was standing before a long metal table with three other medical students one day when I faced my ultimate challenge.

On the table was a long black bag with a zipper running down the middle. In the air around us, assaulting our sinuses, was the sharp chemical smell of formaldehyde. Inside the bag was a dead person—a cadaver.

It had been assigned to our group, and we were expected to dissect it, organ by organ, limb by limb, learning by touch, sight, and firsthand experience the contours, textures, colors, and inner realms of the human body.

I had known this was coming. We all did, and everyone felt some degree of discomfort about this part of our education. The cadaver stage of medical school has been chronicled profusely. Some students name their cadavers—names like Louise, Jim, or Butch. It is a tactic to relieve the discomfort of knowing that before us lies a person who lived life as we do, felt jealousy and fear, and perhaps made art, wrote poetry, raised children and sacrificed for them, decorated Christmas trees, wrapped birthday presents, had been in love and in lust, had had a broken heart.

But beyond all of this, I had to combat another level of discomfort; Navajos do not touch the dead. Ever.

It is one of the strongest rules in our culture. The dead hold *ch'įįndi*s, or evil spirits, that are simply not to be tampered with. When a person dies, the "good" part of the person leaves with the spirit, while the "evil" part stays with the physical body. That belief is so strong that before the advent of mortuaries, Navajos sought out Pueblo Indians, missionaries, white traders, or other outsiders to bury their dead. When a person dies in a hogan, the hogan is destroyed. Sometimes Navajo people nowadays bring their dying relatives to the hospital simply to prevent them from dying in their home. In many other cases hospitals are avoided. Navajo people know that death lies inside hospital walls, and therefore hospitals are filled with *ch'įįndis*.

Many strong superstitions about the dead are woven throughout our beliefs. Sometimes a dead person can become a skinwalker. A young woman from a sheep camp near Farmington above the San Juan River was said to have turned into a skinwalker. A mud clan man from Lukaichukai was made lame after he touched the body of a dead horse, which had also been lame. A healthy man from Tuba City died in his sleep after touching the body of his dead uncle. While there was no shortage of such stories, they were whispered things that I'd caught only in passing conversations between the old people or my aunts or my grandmother and her sister. Mostly these things, thought too terrible, were not discussed. Even speaking the word "death" holds bad karma for a Navajo.

There may have been sound reasons for the Navajo taboo about touching the dead, as there are for the Jewish stricture against eating pork. At the time when the Jewish taboo was set in place, pork often carried the dreaded trichinosis. Dead bodies, too, can be infected with possibly contagious disease. Perhaps long ago an astute Navajo medicine man figured out that touching a corpse might unknowingly spread disease. But whatever the reason, from the earliest age, a Navajo person becomes aware of this aversion. My grandmother and aunts spoke many times of the terrible things that could transpire if someone were to touch or brush against a dead person: things like madness, loss of fertility, death. One who has brushed against a corpse needs to undergo a ceremony (Enemy Way) to purify and release the *ch'įįndi* spirit. It is an elaborate and costly event.

In medical school this taboo confronted me on every level. Never before had I been asked to do anything that directly violated the beliefs of my culture. Had I been more sophisticated, I might have requested some kind of permission from the dean of students to watch instead of touch, on the grounds that it violated my culture. Certain schools today may make allowances or concessions for such a taboo— much of what is learned from dissecting a cadaver can be gotten from books, from 3-D holograph computer programs whose images simulate the human body, or from "virtual" body programs. But at the time I felt that I had no option. If I wanted to become a doctor, I had to dissect.

Standing in front of my cadaver I thought back on stories about this person and that person who had touched a dead thing, and the consequences that befell them.

I thought about all the *ch'įįndi*s of all the dead people around me in that lab room. I looked at the faces of my classmates. They too looked slightly nervous and a little edgy. I think all medical students approach their first cadaver with some trepidation. I wondered if my classmates could read my face and see that I was feeling the bitter taste of fear rising in the back of my throat.

The zipper on the black bag was opened. I looked down, bracing myself.

There below me was an older male of medium build. His skin was shriveled and toughened by formaldehyde, a slate-gray color that I'd never seen on a living person. At first glance, it was revolting and I struggled to quell my nausea. With its lifeless color, the cadaver almost appeared to be a plastic or rubber doll, with shapes that could have been human features at one time, but had ceased to be. Its "non-human" appearance helped me forget that this had once been a real, breathing home for a human soul. I shifted my gaze away from the corpse's face, and leaned hard against the table to still the dizziness.

The experience would have been much worse for a traditional Navajo. After all, I am half *bilagáana* and come from a relatively modern family, and I knew I should set aside these beliefs as superstitions. But even for me the problem arose. As I glanced again at the gray, rubbery form that had once been a man, I thought: *What will happen to me if I do this?*

By this time, my desire to become a doctor was very strong, as I am sure it is for all medical students. We were studying hard, training hard, and had competed against difficult odds just to be admitted to Stanford's halls, which had their own kind of sacredness. There had been more than four thousand applications for our coveted eighty-six spots. At this point, although a part of me was terrified of the next step forward, I knew there was no going back.

Okay, I thought. *This is what I want, the knowledge I will acquire here is like that of a medicine man. I will be able to bring home a tremendous gift. And if I am good enough, my work could even fight processes that cause death. In the course of a career, I could help thousands of my people.*

Cast in this light, my decision became easier. I took a deep breath. Someone handed me a scalpel. *I'm not afraid,* I told myself. *I'm not afraid.* I reached down to the shape below me and slid the scalpel into the skin.

▲▲▲▲

One by one, I conquered the most difficult obstacles of medical school. But each step along the way felt like a step further away from my own people and Native ways. Sometimes I caught myself wondering if the path would take me permanently from Dinetah into another universe, with a completely different set of rules and rites. If I did travel down this path, would I ever find my way home again?

The second two years of med school were spent working in hospital wards where we were taught the basics of clinical medicine in pediatrics, OB-GYN, and psychiatry, as well as in more specialized areas like radiation, cardiology, urology, and surgery.

Right from the beginning I fell in love with surgery. The

instruments lined up on the mayo stand, silver on dark blue cloth, seemed to have a soft, warm glow. Touching and handling them was like picking up sorcerer's wands. Seeing the inside parts of a living human body, watching surgeons open up the body and operate, was just as magical, unlike anything I'd ever experienced. It was both shocking and enchanting. Each body looked very different from every other one, and each person's organs are as unique as their eyes or the shape of their nose.

For a Navajo person, a further element of inhibition was added to this intimate adventure inside another person. Our tribe has a great respect for private, spatial boundaries. Touching another person—especially a person one does not know—is not acceptable. To ask personal questions is just as bad. Yet surgery is a gross invasion of privacy. Moreover, in Navajo society there is respect for others. There is respect for speech. Navajos do not interrupt, as white people do. Yet, a successful surgeon *must* ask the deepest and most probing questions of their patients. It is essential. Too, just as it had been difficult for me to touch the cadaver, so it was also difficult for me to touch the insides of bodies. It went against an instinctual core of my being.

Surgery seemed terrible, but it was also wonderful, because it would do good, could save life.

I believe that surgery is one of the most intimate forms of human contact, closer even than sex. (Probably the only more intimate human act is birthing.) Watching the surgeons at Stanford, I knew with certainty, despite any Navajo cultural objections, that surgery was what I wanted to do. It was the hardest thing in the world—and the most disturbing as a Navajo—but it was where I wanted to be.

But in pursuing surgery my obstacles would be serious. First, I was a woman, and at that time very few women were accepted in surgery programs. Only about 4 percent of practicing surgeons were women. It was extremely competitive.

Second, I was a Native American. To my knowledge there were only a few Native American surgeons in the entire world, and I didn't know any who were women. Also, as I have said, performing surgery went against some important aspects of Navajo philosophy. I would have these huge hurdles to cross before I could make it in the surgical field. The way I got past them had a lot to do with a man named Dr. Ron Lujan.

I was lucky. During my Stanford training I was able to return home to New Mexico for periodic rotations at Acoma-Cañyoncito-Laguna Hospital (ACL) quite near the Navajo reservation. There I met the man who would become my mentor, friend, and colleague, as well as my greatest challenger, Dr. Lujan.

ACL, a bright, new hospital with sparkling equipment, was near Mount Taylor, the southern sacred Navajo mountain, and only thirty miles away from my parents' house. Being there was like being home again.

Over six feet tall (Grandma, whom he had treated from time to time, called him "a tall drink of water"), with dark hair and a graying streak in front, Dr. Lujan was from the Taos and San Juan Pueblo tribes and is an accomplished surgeon. Up until I met him, I had always assumed that there were no Native American surgeons, or that if there were one, he'd probably be one thirty-second Cherokee or some such thing. Ron Lujan was a full-blooded Indian and looked it. When he wasn't with his family, he spent much of his free time on his father's ranch near Taos, working with cattle.

He was widely known simply as Lujan. From the moment I met him, he'd called me (anticipating my future in a way that was encouraging yet somehow disarming) "Doctor." Whenever things got really trying or I came upon a difficult patch in training, I'd call him on the phone. "Lujan?" I'd ask. "Doctor," he'd reply, in his deep, low voice. It was a bit of a joke, since medical students are uniformly uncomfortable with the title up until and even sometimes past the time they get their M.D. Yet he gave it to me unequivocally. I felt it was a challenge, almost a dare.

Lujan worked (and still does) with patients from two small pueblos, Acoma and Laguna, as well as a small satellite Navajo community called Canyoncito. When I first met him, I'd not yet learned how to relate to patients. I was uncomfortable with the whole process of taking histories and performing physicals—I could not get past the sense that I was being rude. Patients' intimate lives and the details about their bodies and illnesses seemed none of my business. I could not help but sense discomfort in an old man, when I, a young woman, reached out to feel his lymph nodes, or opened his shirt to listen to his heart. I would wince as well, it made me so uneasy. But Lujan's bedside manner was gracious and warm. Somehow he—also an Indian—had conquered this dilemma.

To be a good doctor outside of the Native American world would mean probing deeply into a patient's life and history. A good doctor asks a lot of questions and looks searchingly into the patient's eyes, which communicates caring and interest. In the Native American world, this way of behaving is a terrible, embarrassing intrusion. Personal, private information is just like property; disclosing it is a gift, and it is rude to ask for it. Staring into another person's eyes is considered very rude. At Stanford I'd been accused of seeming remote and disinterested, but I had merely been following the Navajo custom of respecting space and avoiding eye contact. At the time it was terribly upsetting, and it made me wonder if I was really cut out for medicine.

Lujan talked effortlessly with everyone, from the hospital CEOs to the janitors. He was intimidated by no one, and he treated everyone the same. He helped me overcome my ingrained reticence to touch and probe. He made me—locked up as I was inside my own world, shy to begin with, and having that natural Navajo reserved personality—see that the doctor-patient relationship could be relaxed and enjoyable. He helped me find ways to overcome the cultural taboos about touching and making eye contact.

Before each examination he would sit and chat with his patients about the weather, horses, cattle, crops, upcoming feast days and dances on the pueblos, and anything else that happened to be going on in the communities surrounding ACL. He often talked about wanting to be at his father's ranch working with the livestock, riding out on the range, finding lost cows, and fixing broken fences. It often seemed that he had as much concern for cattle as for his patients— he would have made an equally wonderful veterinarian—but this put his patients totally at ease. He wasn't invasive in his questions, and through gentle conversation he was able to learn many things he needed to know as a physician. His patients loved him, and he was deeply concerned with their welfare. Sometimes he made house calls along narrow and remote dirt roads, to see patients who had trouble getting to the hospital. His interactions showed me how Indian patients could be cared for by an Indian physician.

Moreover, Lujan felt acutely the losses that our people had historically sustained, and the need to compensate with outstanding care. "They [the Indian people] deserve the best," he'd say. "You need to train to be able to give it to them."

As I watched Lujan speak to his patients about their animals or ask about their relatives, gleaning important medical information and distracting them from the examination process, it all began to click. Suddenly, quite magnificently, everything seemed right about medicine. This was the ideal practice for both physician and patient. I hoped someday to have a surgical practice like Lujan's, and I decided to stay in medicine, in spite of my feelings of extreme discomfort with patients.

Dr. Lujan also took me with him into the OR. This gave me further incalculable experience and later provided me with a definite advantage over the other Stanford students. He operated at Cibola General Hospital in Grants, New Mexico, about twenty miles west of ACL. Oftentimes over the years Lujan and I would be the only physicians present in the OR—he as primary surgeon, and I as first assistant. Our nurse anesthetist was Eddie Sanshu, an Indian from Laguna, and sometimes our nurses were Acoma or Laguna Indians as well. As we brought in our Indian patients for surgery I felt we were making history—we had established an all-Indian surgical team! It seemed extraordinary. Indian people were treating Indian people without a white man in sight. The hope of replicating this accomplishment in my own operating room would sustain me in the years that followed.

Yet, at first, Lujan tried to talk me out of becoming a surgeon. Over and over I learned that the field of surgery exacted a price that was often formidable. By assigning me patients with complicated problems, Lujan made sure I knew this, and when I was very new on his team, he sent me difficult patients. He was testing me.

Once at ACL he sent me into an examining room where I encountered a middle-aged Navajo man sitting on a chair. His right leg was exposed and nearly twice the size of his left. The skin beneath the knee was gnarled and thickened like tree bark. Midway down the calf was a wound, about five by five inches. The skin was gone, and the wound penetrated to the muscle layer. Tiny insects crawled in and out. Sickened by the sight and smell of the wound, I excused myself and fled to the hallway. Lujan was waiting for me by the nurses' station, his eyes full of laughter. "Well, Doctor, what is your diagnosis?" I was so nauseated I couldn't speak.

"Still want to be a doctor?" he asked, smiling. Then his voice turned serious: "Mr. Blackgoat has lymphedema from an old injury to the leg. The fluid from the leg doesn't drain properly into the rest of the body, so it just stays there, and the leg swells up. Eventually it puts so much pressure on the skin that it starts to break and form ulcers. Those insects, by the way, are maggots." I must have looked stunned, because he smiled again. "Don't worry, Doctor, they're actually doing him a favor. If you noticed, that wound is very clean—because the maggots only eat dead skin and tissue. They leave living healthy tissue alone. He needs to be admitted and I want you to clean that leg up. Peroxide will kill 'em."

I went and got a large basin, the peroxide, and some dressing supplies, as Lujan smiled away.

"Mr. Blackgoat, I'm going to clean up your leg, okay?" I said timidly when I returned to the room. I positioned his foot in the basin and poured peroxide over the wound. Almost instantly, the stream of peroxide lifted off the creatures and carried them into the basin. Only a few remained, which I extracted with a forceps. I dumped the basin out, rinsed the leg again, and wrapped the wound with a sterile dressing. "We'll get you into the hospital for a few days to take care of that," I said. I walked out of the room to the nurses' station. "All done," I said to Lujan with a level gaze. He looked at me, and I thought I caught a glimpse of respect in his eyes. "Let's go make rounds, Doctor," he said.

Cleaning up Mr. Blackgoat's leg was only one of many little challenges that Lujan threw at me over the months. He knew that at the Stanford surgery program, I would be grilled by the surgeons, so in preparation he began to question me, too.

"Define the borders of Hesselbach's triangle," he asked me.

"What are Clark's levels of melanoma?"

"How about Breslow's?"

"Name the Duke's stages of colon cancer."

"Who was Theodor Kocher?"

As we rounded, he fired away at me. I often got frustrated and even angry. Sometimes I wanted to snap back: "Enough already!"

Later, when I went back to Stanford to do my rotation in general surgery, I thanked him. He put me way ahead of the game. He had exposed me to many of the questions I was

asked. I'd already seen and assisted on many of the procedures we were trained to do. The result was that I made a fa-
vorable impression on my professors, and high grades, which
eventually added up.

From Lujan, too, I learned another invaluable lesson
about what I would encounter as a surgeon. "As a minority
physician, you will be constantly challenged," he said. "Your
decisions will be questioned, your authority doubted. To be
successful, you will have to have higher standards than
everyone else. You will have to study harder, train longer, and
know your materials backward and forward. In the operating
room, you will need to know the anatomy, how to do the operation, and what alternative operations might also work. You
will have to be prepared to handle any emergency that might
arise."

Time after time in the years to come, I would encounter
skepticism about my abilities. Even after taking all the same
classes, passing all the same tests, and meeting the same requirements for graduation as everyone else, I would be eyed
sideways and doubted at times. My being a surgeon would be
attributed to quota filling, not to the result of hard work and
my own merit. I would always think of his words when this
happened.

Working with Lujan also helped prepare me for the residency position in surgery into which I was accepted.

When I learned I was accepted into the surgery training
program at Stanford, I considered myself fortunate beyond
all possible hope. Many such teaching programs around the
country have only one or two women in an entire group of
residents. Stanford was different. In general surgery it had
four positions available for entering residents, and every year
one or two of those positions were granted to women. Midway through my own residency, that number was increased to
five. The increase was the direct result of our chairman of
surgery, Dr. John Collins, who had a gruff persona and sometimes had a temper. He could be quite intimidating, but due

to his efforts, the year before I entered the program, three women were admitted within one year. According to Stanford folklore, Dr. Collins had been criticized by some of the other surgical program directors. "You're crazy," they told him—crazy for making it easier for woman to enter the field! I would later learn that Dr. Collins cared about many of the same things I did.

At that time there was a distinct and powerful perception in the national surgical community that women were not suited to general surgery. General surgery was considered the hardest residency and was a prerequisite to further surgical training for cardiac surgery, neurosurgery, and plastic surgery. Mastering general surgery requires mental toughness and physical stamina, along with tremendous self-discipline.

But it didn't matter what anyone said—Dr. Collins stuck with his commitment to integrate women into the field. And so, for a woman who wanted to be a surgeon, Stanford was one of the best places to be. My colleagues and the attending surgeons didn't treat us any differently from our male counterparts. Our proportion later approached 30 percent—not much different from medical school. (Now the proportion is almost 50 percent.)

Actually, racism was much less of an issue in med school than in the rest of the world. It didn't matter what race or social class you came from—your standing in the med school system was what counted. Interns were above first- and second-year med students, residents were above interns, doctors were above all—the internal ranking system canceled out all outside social hierarchies. As students progressed through it, we earned the respect of our standing at each higher rung. It was a true merit system. In fact, few people even asked me anything about myself. With the exception of a handful of surgeons, most did not mention my Navajo background, if they even knew about it. Dr. Collins appreciated the Navajo culture, and I gave him a beautiful Navajo rug at the end of my training. His wife told me he was deeply moved by his "Ganado Red." This idea of him moved by something, when he often seemed so remote, was deeply touching.

Dr. Collins wasn't the only doctor who displayed a love for Indian culture. Dr. Don Nagel, an orthopedist with whom I worked in my surgery program, had a whole collection of Navajo rugs. Dr. Francis Marzoni, from the Palo Alto clinic, told me he was an avid Tony Hillerman reader. Once, when I dropped something off at the office of Dr. Craig Miller, a well-known cardiac surgeon, I noticed that he had posters of Native Americans on his walls. The next time I met him, I said: "I see you have pictures of my relatives on your walls." A look of complete surprise and puzzlement passed over his face, until he realized I was teasing him.

In general, I didn't discuss my background with people at Stanford, and many of them didn't know I was Navajo. I came from a separate world, a world I thought they could never understand. I focused on skills that would help me become successful in the white world. I learned how to communicate. And the longer I stayed outside the sacred mountains the more I adopted "white" behavior. I felt I was losing touch with my culture, and inside I mourned this loss.

▲▲▲▲

In January 1987, during my rotation at Santa Clara Valley Medical Center, considered by residents to be one of our most difficult rotations, I had a major setback.

It was the year of the famous Libby Zion case at New York Hospital, in which an overworked resident had made mistakes that led to the death of the daughter of Sidney Zion, a prominent New York journalist. What happened to me was comparable in that an overworked resident almost caused a death. But in this case both the resident and the patient were the same person: me.

We worked sixteen hours a day on regular days and sometimes thirty-six hours straight during on-call days, which was every third or fourth night. This became physically, mentally, and emotionally exhausting. The combination of sleep deprivation and dealing with serious illness and injury was having its effect on us. The drive to the valley took over thirty minutes and while I was in training, one resident had several accidents, caused by falling asleep at the wheel when driving home. The effect on me was different: I began to have fevers. They sometimes took my temperature as high as 103, accompanied by chills and mild flank pain.

My roommate Carol Kemper examined me, drew blood cultures and a complete blood count, and took a urine sample. "Probably pyelonephritis," she said, a kidney infection. But there was no sign of infection in my urinalysis, and my pain went away. The second day I was sick was a Friday, and I was to be on call on Saturday. I was thoroughly drained, alternately sweating during the fevers and huddling beneath blankets through the chills, but I could not find anyone to cover my shift for me.

We'd all heard stories about residents working when they were sick and getting fluids or antibiotics through IVs. It was part of the unwritten code of toughness and machismo that we were supposed to live by, proving ourselves to be surgeon material. Many surgery programs had used this same code as a reason not to train women, something similar to the military attitude. It was felt that women couldn't handle the training. So I knew I had to live up to the code.

Somehow I made it through Saturday night working. My first day back at Stanford was a Sunday, and I was on call again. Ellen Mahoney, my chief resident, could tell I was not at all well. "I'll take care of things and call you if I need you," she said. She sent me to rest in the call rooms. I went up, plugged in an IV bag, and collapsed on the couch.

That evening in the hallway I passed another resident in the halls. "Lori?" he asked. I turned around. "Is your name also Janette? Janette Lorraine Cupp?"

I nodded.

"I was reviewing your blood cultures in the lab today," he said. "They're positive for staph." I had just walked past the ER. I immediately turned around, went back, and checked myself in.

It turned out I had an infected fluid collection lying between my lung and the chest wall, a "pleural effusion." The infection had broken through the wall of my lung and invaded my chest cavity, forming an empyema, which had to be drained with a chest tube. As my family came in from New Mexico, I was fighting for my life.

Lujan, hearing of my condition from my family, kept track of my illness through calls to my doctors. Our conversations often ended with his words of encouragement and a "Keep your head up, Doctor."

Carol had dug up a bunch of papers on my condition but it was a good thing she didn't tell me what she found: Back then, in 1987, 30 percent of young patients with staphylococcus pneumonia died. It took ten days before my fever finally broke. In all I spent three weeks in the hospital at Stanford and another three on bedrest and antibiotic pills.

I will never forget the care I received when I was sick at Stanford. In some ways it was the best and most important part of my education, because I learned what it is like to be on the other side of our profession, as a very sick patient.

I noticed things no doctor would ever notice—such as the fact that the hallways were cleaned by large noisy machines in the middle of the night; my roommate would change every few days and another patient and all their relatives would appear, just a curtain away; strangers were constantly coming into my room, unannounced, without introducing themselves, and physically probing my body. Their hands prodded my body. Doctors and nurses gazed into my eyes, and for the first time I was profoundly aware of the experience of a Navajo person in the medical system.

For me, being sick served an unbelievably important purpose in medical school. It taught me what it was like to be the patient and see through a patient's eyes. I would never forget that lesson. I never saw medicine in the same way again.

Later, after I left Stanford, a new system was created to provide coverage for sick residents there. Today, when one resident falls sick, another from one of the less busy services is pulled from service and is assigned cross-coverage. But perhaps it was not the residency call system that had caused my illness at all. As a resident, I had violated the basic Navajo principles of living in harmony and balance. My life was completely unbalanced—the long hours, minimal sleep, poor eating habits, and constant stress had taken their toll. It was so ironic; the profession that advocated preventive medicine and a healthy lifestyle ignored those principles when it came to those they trained, and how they cared for themselves.

A few months later I was back home in New Mexico, recovering. Lujan brought me a gift: a yellow stone bear with turquoise eyes. Was it something he gave me for protection? I thought of the Navajo story of the woman and the bear, how she put the bear's body on her own, how she climbed inside it and was safe and strong and ready for anything she might encounter next.

The year of my chief residency, the Native American students at Stanford performed an Honor Dance for me at the annual Stanford powwow. It was a gorgeous, warm summer day. I wore a blue velvet dress with silver buttons and as the drums beat, I walked around a circle and felt my moccasins pad on the soft green grass of the campus. Following me were many of the Native American Stanford students and my other colleagues.

I was a surgeon. My sister and friends were watching me, and so was my grandmother, who had traveled all the way from New Mexico, her eyes bright. It was the first time I'd ever been honored by a Native community. My heart was filled with emotion.

I was finished with my training, and it would soon be time to go back home to Dinetah and begin my practice. I quickly joined the Indian Health Service (IHS) and requested a job among the *Diné*. After some negotiation, the Indian hospital in Gallup, New Mexico, hired me. Gallup was a quick fifty miles from Crownpoint, my hometown.

Home, I thought. *I am going home again.*

Chapter Four

▲▲▲▲

LIFE OUT OF BALANCE

*People have power to upset the Circle of Life.
We have made weapons that kill more game
than we need. We have farmed land that
should have been left wild. We have dug
ditches and built dams. All these things have
changed the life around us, and in the end
have changed us too.*

—GEORGE BLUEEYES,
Navajo medicine man

Hello, I am Dr. Cupp, your surgeon," I would
say, holding out a hand to shake. But very often my
hand would remain there, suspended in air for a
long, strange, uncomfortable moment, ungrasped.
Then, when the hand did clasp, there was no firm-
ness in the grip, the way there is when *bilagáana*s
shake. It was pressureless. Delicate.

"I am Navajo," I'd continue. "My clans are
Tsi'naajinii and *Ashįįhi Dineé*. My grandmother
is from White Horse Lake." Yes, my patients
would say, they had heard of my grandmother,
they knew my clans, and the older ones would peer
at me curiously. Sometimes they would ask, "You
are . . . Navajo?"

My heart would sink.

In medical school I had learned about the Krebs

cycle. I had learned to perform laparoscopic surgery and had helped open the chambers of a human heart. But in doing so, I had acquired many white mannerisms. With my short, pageboy-styled hair and white medical jacket and a stethoscope around my neck I did not look like a *Diné* woman to my *Diné* patients. The cost of my knowledge had been high. I still had much to learn, and much to unlearn.

Although I always knew I'd come home, I had not known what it would be like. I thought home would feel like a pair of old, worn-in moccasins, perfectly molded to the shape of my feet, that I could slip back into. I thought *Dinétah* and I would always be a perfect fit—instantly and instinctually right, the way that the air, dry and clean, scented with piñon and wood smoke, always smells right to me. But when I finished my education and returned home, I found that in many ways coming back to the reservation was as hard as leaving it had been.

After I finished my education in surgery, I began a new battle. The Indian Health Service wanted to send me to Oklahoma, but I insisted that I be allowed to work at home. It didn't make sense for a Navajo to work with Cherokees, I argued, and in the end, they agreed. So I got my dream job. It was exactly what I wanted to be doing, exactly where I wanted to be: working as a surgeon at the Gallup Indian Medical Center (GIMC), an IHS hospital that served the Navajo reservation and surrounding area.

Gallup was a reservation border town, that nestled among the red and white rock ridges and spilled into the valleys of the westernmost part of New Mexico. I bought a small house on the edge of town, at the base of an outcrop of dramatic white rock in the Hogback Mountains, what Navajos call Tsé yik'ááń. My home had beautiful gray-blue carpeting and a fireplace in the central room. A skylight let in muted white daylight from the ceiling.

My companions—two cairn terriers, one named Bouncer and the other Shush, the Navajo word for "bear"—loved the

yard and surrounding desert. But perhaps best, my grandmother Grace soon moved from my mother's house to live
with me. I set her up in her own room. In the distance, visible from Grandma's window, a sculptured finger of rock
called Churchrock pointed up at the enormous bowl of the
sky, as if to emphasize the grace of the land and the blue
infinity above it. The community that lies in the shadow of
that pointing digit was where Grace was born in a hogan
ninety years before. Her relatives live there to this day, and
Grace often visited her sister Janice in a small house, filled
with photographs of weddings and newborns, blue squares of
elementary school pictures, and other family memorabilia.
Farther still, but in clear view from just down the road or
atop the nearby hill that she loved to climb, was Tsoodził, or
Mount Taylor, the southern sacred mountain.

In the creation stories Tsoodził was fastened to the earth
with a stone knife. It was covered with turquoise blankets
and decorated with dark mists and female rain. Dootl'-
izhii At'eed (Turquoise Girl) was sent to live there, and Big
Snake was sent to guard the doorway. It is a very holy place and
to live within view of it is a blessing. From the moment I saw
it, I knew Grandmother would love our new home, as I did.

The house was simple but just right for us. One of the best
features of the area was that when it rained, the rain made a
waterfall that cascaded dramatically down the nearby cliffs.
There were nice long walks to take into tiny secret canyons
amidst the hills. Grandma would walk each afternoon, with a
big stick, along the rims and valleys with the dogs. Sometimes she would come back with her arms full of flowers,
which she boiled into a delicious tea that eased her aches
and pains. From that house, in a matter of minutes, I could
drive to the hospital when my beeper buzzed.

This was where I was supposed to be. I was coming home
richer than I had left, laden with gifts, knowledge, and
state-of-the-art medical training. It was now time for me to

give back to the people who have given me the opportunity to pursue my education—my tribe had footed much of the Dartmouth bill.

Atop Gallup's highest promontory stands the Gallup Indian Medical Center. The blue-and-white five-story hospital, with its wide halls and large, low windows, is characteristic of buildings the government built in the 1960s. It commands an impressive eagle's-nest view of the surrounding hills and the rust-colored bay of desert below. Like all Indian Health Service facilities, GIMC treats exclusively Native people, mostly Navajo, although some patients come from Zuni, Hopi, and other Indian pueblos.

All of the medicine practiced at IHS hospitals like GIMC is free to Indian patients, as a result of treaties between the U.S. government and Native American tribes. Sometimes people say they think that is an enormous benefit, proof that Native people are treated well in this country. As I grew accustomed to my new practice in Gallup, it often occurred to me that much of what we were treating were white men's diseases—syndromes and conditions the people would never have known if not for the European colonizers. I am referring to much more than the infamous smallpox-infected blankets. There were other diseases—tuberculosis, measles, whooping cough, and mumps. These and the malaria, yellow fever, and influenza brought by Columbus, had killed off 90 percent of all Native Americans in the New World. Still other diseases were caused by lifestyle changes, such as poor diet and inactivity—an indirect result of the influence of acculturation.

The ancestors of my people who migrated across the expanses of desert and mountain of the Southwest had rarely suffered from obesity, diabetes, or heart disease. Traditional life required a vigorous physical lifestyle, and was highly protective against these diseases. Smoking-related diseases—hypertension, heart disease, lung cancer, oral cancers—did not exist either. Tobacco was used rarely and in moderation, kept in "balance." Just as many of the diseases were Western diseases, the medicine we were practicing was Western medicine, practiced in the white men's way—and the patients knew it. It seemed to me sometimes that the whole arrangement was an awkward fit.

The doctors at GIMC found their Navajo patients both confusing and compelling. Many of them worked through translators and often after their conditions were explained to them through these translators, the patients still did not seem to have a clue what was going on. And vice versa: the physicians didn't really understand the words of their patients.

These doctors told incredible stories about their cases. Tim Simpson, the chief surgeon on GIMC's staff, was a British doctor who had worked for the IHS in Gallup and at Chinle for several years. One night he invited me over for dinner with his wife, and told me the story of a patient of his, a middle-aged man upon whom he'd operated to repair a perforation of the intestine. "Inside my patient I made a remarkable finding," he said. "A two-and-a-half-centimeter porcupine quill was lodged inside the large intestine. It had ruptured and was causing internal bleeding," Tim said with incredulity.

"The chap was of the firm belief that he'd been witched," he said, raising an eyebrow. The patient had told Tim that an enemy had placed the porcupine quill in his abdomen. "Truth is," Tim said, "it's pretty damn hard to find an explanation for how that quill got in there." When asked, Tim said, the patient swore he had not eaten a porcupine.

Many other patients and cases were equally baffling. One night when I was on duty, soon after I'd begun practicing at GIMC, a man was brought into the intensive care unit.

"Thirty-three-year-old male, status post assault, stab wounds to the back," I noted in my report, adding that he was drunk on arrival and that his workup had revealed a compression

fracture of the thoracic spine. The man's pelvic bone, fortu-
nately, had protected his body from the stabbings. *This is
your lucky day, no serious injury to your spinal cord.* I had
then thought sadly, *You will live to drink again.* The fact
that so many patients showed up intoxicated was depressing
to me.

I went through my usual questionnaire for past medical
history. "Any previous surgery?" I asked.

"No."

"Any major medical problems?"

"No."

"See a doctor on a regular basis?"

"No." Then he sat straight up, which must have caused
him incredible pain, and said, "Hey, this thing in my nose is
bothering me!"

"Sorry, we need that tube in for a while. It's draining your
stomach." My questioning went on. When I came to the
family history questions, I asked, "Any diseases run in your
family?"

"No, but my dad died of choking to death. So did my
brother."

Stunned for a moment, I was silent, then tentatively
asked, "How did they choke?"

"The skinwalkers did it," he said, lowering his voice, as if
afraid someone might hear him. "They both choked on
pieces of food. My brother died first, in January 1988, then
my dad in January 1989."

I tried to remember if I had ever heard of anything like
this in the medical literature. At the same time the stories I
was told when I was little came rushing back at me. Skinwalkers. Goose bumps rose on my arms. Skinwalkers were
the face of evil in Navajo country. They were supposed to
practice witchcraft, using pieces of a person's body—hair,
fingernail parings, whatever they could find that belonged to
the victim—to turn their magic against them. In the ghost
stories of my childhood, skinwalkers could be hitchhikers in

the backseat of the car one moment and human wolves the next. It was also said that these wolves ran alongside pickup trucks at night, trying to enter through the windows. I shuddered involuntarily, brushed by these memories like a cold breeze.

"So where are you from?" I asked, trying to bring my scientific mind into play and thinking maybe geography would offer some clues to this man's story.

"Sheepsprings," the man said.

"Lots of skinwalkers around there?"

"Well," the man said, "we think my ex-wife may have had something to do with it."

He was hedging. He didn't want to come right out and say she was a skinwalker, but he clearly thought she either was one, or knew one. At the same time I tried like mad to think of a disease this choking could be attributed to: a neurological disorder? A muscular disease? But I was also curious: was choking to death a murder typical of skinwalkers?

Stories of skinwalkers, ghosts, and bad spirits, people who had not followed the Beauty Way, now became a regular part of my clinic experiences. It was my initiation into the world of medicine on the rez. The unusual intersection of peoples and lifestyles meant that I would see and hear things that were not described in textbooks or encountered anywhere else in the world. Inside our Navajo patients we would come across unforgettable things like the porcupine quill. The place where I was to work was thus medically unique and interesting right from the start.

On one occasion I saw something few surgeons will ever see. Peter Tempest, a colleague and fellow surgeon, had an interesting case scheduled for the OR, and in the absence of another surgeon to assist him one of our best Navajo OR nurses, Marge Cleveland, was helping out. I was weak and exhausted from working all night the night before, but decided to check in to see how he was doing. "Need me in here?" I asked, poking my head through the swinging doors.

Peter had his patient's abdomen opened and was bending over him, peering inside.

"Check it out!" He waved me over.

I went to scrub, and once I was gloved and gowned, I came back. Peter pointed to the lit-up CT scans: "Do you see the pelvic alien?" On the screen was a cluster of what looked like dark eggs, buried amid the patient's organs.

"I just found another nest. There are literally hundreds of cysts in here." I came over to the operating table. "Marge and I have just discovered something."

Marge moved to the side, and I took the clamps that held open the abdomen. To get at the cysts, Peter was burning through a layer of adhesions. "Look at this," he said.

As I peered into the opened abdominal cavity, right in the pelvic region, I saw a huge, shiny, round object. Another sidled against the liver. But the one that Peter pointed at, next to the spleen, was even more impressive. It was the size of a softball, only more irregular, white, and dense.

"Can you believe it?"

"Pretty wild." I'd seen a smaller echinococcal cyst like this in a specimen bottle when I was a resident. The large ones are referred to as "mother" cysts. If they burst, they send out numerous smaller "daughter" cysts that implant themselves and begin to grow. After a while they become "mothers" themselves. It really is like an alien invasion.

"Call Dr. Tempest and Dr. Iralu," Peter told a nurse. "I want them to see this." Dr. Iralu was our infectious disease specialist, and Dr. Tempest was Peter's father, a senior physician at the hospital.

"I always wanted my parents to see what I do, too," I said, teasingly.

"Well, I don't want him to think I'm a slacker," Peter said.

When Drs. Tempest and Iralu came in, Peter held up the newly extracted, enormous, hard white cyst, cupped in his hands like a shiny planet, and delivered the news that an even larger one that we had not yet removed lay beneath. In addition the "pelvic alien" was troublesome because it had become connected by a sinus tract to the patient's ureter. And multitudes of smaller white cystic pockets freckled the dark insides of his abdomen.

"Echinococcus," the elder Dr. Tempest said, confirming the diagnosis. "A parasite that cycles between sheep and sheepdogs. People get mixed up in it where there's a lot of contact."

"What are you going to do for him?" asked Dr. Iralu. He stood on a stool, looking into the opened abdomen with awe.

"Try to get out a few of these major ones, do something about the sinus tract from the ureter, and close him back up. We could never get all of them out."

Echinococcus is very rare in the rest of the United States, but because Navajos often live very close to their animals, it is occasionally seen at GIMC. Still, no one in the room had ever seen a case as bad as that of this forty-three-year-old man who also had relatives with the disease. The nurses placed the cysts in labeled specimen jars, where they sank to the bottom and seemed to stare out at us like a collection of white eyes. Peter's patient would be given Albendazole, a drug that combats the parasite. But unless something was done to disinfect the animals and treat the other infected people, it would probably come back in a chronic form again. The parasite had invaded a remote community of human beings, where it was obviously making itself quite at home, loading their bodies with its offspring.

▲▲▲▲

As I learned the ropes I also noticed the unique culture of the hospital itself. The higher positions in the GIMC administration were almost all held by Anglos. The entire medical staff—with the exception of Dr. Taylor McKenzie, who was the first Navajo doctor; Dr. Valden Johnson, a Navajo anesthesiologist; and I—were non-Navajo. Roy Smith, a Navajo from Standing Rock, was our patient advocate. A strong and stocky man, with a ponytail protruding from beneath his baseball cap, Roy found ways for families to help sick members get around, arranged for rehabilitation, worked out finances, and even helped them deal with the one thing that Navajos can't stand to think about—advance directives, or living wills.

Because Navajos are so uncomfortable with death and dying, speaking to them about making a decision to end life, to stop a life-support system, was nearly impossible and had to be handled very carefully. The discomfort arises partly because of the Navajo belief in the power of language, the belief that you can "speak" something into existence. Most Navajos, for instance, would never say, "If I fall into a coma, I don't want to be kept alive." Such verbalizing would be seen as asking for it to happen.

Roy was able to finesse these problematic and culturally sensitive areas with skill and kindness. Patients responded well to his presence. And he handled the *bilagáana* administrators well, too. He was quite a talented man.

As for Dr. McKenzie, I had grown up in awe of him. He had been in practice on the rez when I was a child, and everyone knew of him. By the time I came to GIMC, however, he was nearing retirement. He rarely worked in the OR and mostly did clinic visits and a few special cases.

When I first got to GIMC I often observed Roy, Dr. McKenzie, and Valden Johnson, who was near my own age. We had our own silent code of medicine. Sometimes when we saw a brash young Anglo doctor whip through an exam gazing inappropriately, hurrying, talking loudly, cutting off the patient when they ventured to ask a question, and moving their hands over their bodies in a methodical, impersonal, irreverent fashion, we exchanged glances. I saw my own unease echoed in Roy's eyes. That was not the way to treat a Navajo person, not if you wanted the patient to respond positively, not if you wanted them to get well.

One afternoon, while removing an infected gallbladder with a colleague, Barney Nelson, I grew extremely frustrated. Cast in the blue glow of the video monitor, Barney was suctioning up a mauve pool of bile and blood in the area where we were working, while I removed the gallbladder and brought it up through a small incision in the abdomen. It was a laparoscopic procedure, in which tiny tools are used through a "keyhole" incision in the abdomen, at that time a state-of-the-art technology that I'd learned at Stanford.

The patient, a woman in her fifties named Evelyn Bitsui, had come into the hospital for gallbladder surgery. She'd arrived with her daughter, Josephine Smith, who translated for her. When I met them, Evelyn was lying on a hospital bed, waiting for her pre-op consultation. Josephine was seated beside her. Unfortunately Sue Stuart, her surgeon, had come down with the flu.

"Your doctor is sick, Evelyn," I told her. "If you want, I can perform your surgery instead of her, or you can wait and come back another day."

I waited while Josephine translated. They had traveled a long way, perhaps with some trouble, over very muddy roads, the result of hard rains the night before. It would be difficult for them just to leave and come back another day. "Think about it, and I'll come back and see you in a little while," I said.

I was called down to the OR for my first case of the day, a teenage boy who was having increasingly severe attacks of abdominal pain, caused by gallstones. Although he showed no signs of infection, he was in a lot of pain. He looked so uncomfortable, I had scheduled him as early as possible. The surgery was uneventful, and we were finished by nine o'clock.

Then I went over to 2 East, where patients are prepared for surgery, and met up with Evelyn and her daughter. Josephine was clearly worried about her mother. A deep gullied frown lay between her eyebrows, and she kept her hand on her mother's shoulder as she searched my face, as if trying to determine whether to trust me. Josephine was dressed in jeans and an Arizona State University T-shirt, but her mother's clothes, folded on her lap, were traditional: a long cotton print skirt, a matching shirt, and a pile of turquoise necklaces and bracelets. She had worn her best jewelry.

"Momma says she wants to get it over with," Josephine said.

"That's fine," I said, and smiled at her mother. I took a look at her chart. She had a past history of hypertension, back surgery, and left leg sciatica (pain caused by the sciatic nerve, which travels down the back of the leg).

Not bad for sixty years old, I thought. Evelyn was wheeled into the OR, and preparations for her surgery and anesthesia were begun. While Barney and I scrubbed up, Beth Jones, one of our nurse anesthetists, put her to sleep.

A few minutes later, when we first looked into the abdominal cavity with the laparoscope, I saw that we were in for a struggle. The gallbladder was covered with omental adhesions (fatty tissues that are attached to the stomach and colon, which frequently wrap around areas of infection and act as a defense mechanism to control and prevent the infection's spread). Often such adhesions are firmly attached to the gallbladder, so removing them can cause bleeding, which is exactly what happened as I tried to gently release Evelyn's. At first the blood squeezed out slowly from a few spots, then it flowed more heavily. It began along the edges of the omentum and became a miniwaterfall.

Barney and I controlled the bleeding, but not before the operative field was smeared with blood.

"Damn, I can't stand the sight of blood," I said. Barney laughed and handed me a suction irrigator, which washes the area with saline and suctions it back out, so we could proceed with the operation.

Ideally surgeons operate in a "bloodless field," and the very presence of blood indicates that an operation is not going smoothly. Uncontrolled bleeding is a surgical nightmare and can be life threatening. Nowadays we have many ways to stop it, and such situations are fairly rare.

Once the blood was gone, I got a fresh look at the gallbladder. It was inflamed, which made the walls thicker and harder to dissect.

I was tired, it was my third day in a row on call, my feet hurt, and under my gown and gloves, I felt very hot. The new scrub nurse, who was training for this kind of surgery, often handed us the wrong instrument or couldn't locate what we asked for at all. I was beginning to wish I hadn't volunteered to take the case.

"Not that," I snapped at the nurse at one point, and pointed with my nose at a Maryland dissector, which lay on the table beside her. "*That.*"

A few minutes later she handed me another wrong instrument. This time Marge Cleveland, the seasoned OR nurse, intervened. "Not that clamp. *That* one, the toothed grasping forceps," she said.

"I know," said the nurse in an irritated tone, handing me yet another wrong instrument.

"That's still the wrong one. Now watch it—watch it! Don't twist the end of that cable!" I said.

"I *know* that." The new nurse, a woman in her late twenties, had an edge of anger in her voice.

I located the cystic artery, dissected it free, placed metal clips on it, and divided it with miniature scissors. Then I stopped and stared at the video screen. The end of the artery had started bleeding heavily.

I took a deep breath and exhaled. I tried to suction the blood away, but nothing happened. It wasn't working. The suction system had become clogged somewhere.

"I need a bulb syringe right now," I ordered. The nurse scrambled to find one. Meanwhile I considered the possibilities: the surgical clip could have misfired from the "gun"; there might be a small posterior branching vessel that the clip had not closed around; or the vessel might have torn where the clip was placed. These possible explanations were flashing through my mind as I waited for the bulb syringe, which I needed to flush the suction tubing. When I looked up and saw that the nurse still didn't have the suction, I became angry. The blood was slowly rising and had covered the artery.

"Get one *now!*" I shouted this time, realizing that she had totally missed the fact that we were facing an emergency.

Once the suction was working again, I cleared the area of the accumulated blood. As Barney held up the end of the artery with his forceps, I placed another clip slightly lower than the first.

Yes, I thought. *That's it.* The vessel stopped bleeding.

I'd been holding my breath. I exhaled and took a gulp of fresh air. *Calm down, calm down,* I thought, peripherally aware that a combination of things—the heat of the room, my aching feet, the difficulty of the case, and the length of time I'd been operating that morning—was making even small things annoy me. As the rest of the operation refused to proceed smoothly, I found myself growling and swearing. We struggled to dissect through an inflamed plane of tissue between the wall of the gallbladder and the liver, finally freeing the gallbladder, only to encounter another struggle in bringing it out of the abdomen. I felt really hot and lightheaded. But finally, the operation was over.

Evelyn had done just fine, her vital signs had registered normal throughout, and she came out of anesthesia with no difficulty. She had not lost anywhere near enough blood to necessitate a transfusion. *Everything will be fine,* I thought. *Thank God.* Instinctively, I touched my silver bear fetish and felt its smooth, comforting shape.

But everything was not fine. Sometime during the next day, our patient had a stroke.

I will never forget the expressions of pure bewilderment on

the faces of the family of Evelyn Bitsui as they stationed themselves outside the intensive care unit. Sitting in the plastic chairs in an alcove designed for temporary visitors, they held a twenty-four-hour vigil over the next few days. They brought in blankets and food and sometimes it seemed like a little campsite—the only thing missing were the tents and fires. The hours passed, the staff came and went, we had our showers, changed our clothes, ate our dinners, and slept in our own beds. But Josephine Smith, now joined by her son and husband and a small child, who must have been Evelyn's grandson, just stayed right there. They spoke to one another quietly, and each time we left the ICU, they looked up at our faces, searching for clues about Evelyn's condition.

The stroke had partially paralyzed her left side, and she had trouble breathing. For a few days she required a ventilator. When I came to speak with her, her eyes looked unfocused, and she didn't respond to my greeting or questions. It was as though she were looking right past me, at a spot somewhere over my right shoulder. She was staring so intensely, I was tempted on several occasions to turn around and see who was there. She looked right past the members of her family, too. She seemed completely unaware of their presence at her bedside.

Her children remarked that something like this had happened many years before, after her back surgery, which had left her left leg mildly weakened. Upon hearing this, we requested that details of her previous surgery be forwarded from Albuquerque. When the envelope arrived, I pored over the records and shook my head.

In spite of the computer age, physicians in the United States still do not have easy access to medical records from other hospitals, and they are often not requested unless something seems unusual. Although we knew that Evelyn had had surgery years before, neither the patient nor her family had told us that a stroke had been suspected at that time. Her head CT scan had been normal back then, but this time that was not the case—the CT showed an area of infarction to the brain. The lack of blood flow had occurred in the right middle cerebral artery in the temporal parietal region, the area that controls movement of the left arm and leg.

I felt a growing unease. The medical team did a variety of tests to look for the cause of the stroke: an ultrasound of the carotid arteries in the neck, probing for narrowing, damage to the artery walls, and blood clots, and an ultrasound of the heart, looking for abnormalities that might have caused it to develop clots and send them shooting up to the brain. Lastly, Evelyn's blood was tested to check for conditions that would make it thicken and clot easily. Every one of these studies came up normal. It was a mystery. According to all our data, there was no reason for this woman to have had a stroke. She would stay in the hospital for a week so we could assess the damage and then be discharged with a referral to a rehabilitation clinic. She might still recover a lot of her movement, but there was no way to tell just yet.

"No good deed goes unpunished," I said to Tim, using one of his famous quips and wishing, for the hundredth time, that I'd never offered to do that operation.

"That's right," he said wisely. "Remember that."

As I joked with him, an important realization dawned. I could not tell which physiological processes had conspired to bring about Evelyn's stroke, yet instinctively I knew the reason for it. This was not the "doctor" side of me. It was not the white side of me. It was the Navajo. In the pit of my stomach I knew what had happened.

Ever since I finished my surgical training, I had been developing a set of ideas about how to care for patients. The concepts I was beginning to form were bicultural, drawing heavily on a philosophy that is in essence very Navajo. To this day I keep adding to this theory and fine-tuning it. It has to do with working *with* patients to create a superior system of healing.

When I first returned to the Navajo area to work, I realized that although I had been well trained as a surgeon to perform operations, I had received minimal training in how to communicate well with patients. Evelyn was a perfect example. Evelyn had been frightened. I was not the doctor she'd known and was comfortable with. And during her surgery there'd been arguments in the OR. The new nurse assistant had not been listening, and I'd grown angry. The combination of all these variables—my anger, the nurse's inattentive and defensive posture, and Evelyn Bitsui's fear—had been a perfect setup for the complications that had arisen.

My anger had frightened me. Despite all I'd learned in medical school and during residency, a part of me remained underdeveloped. I could be quick-tempered and intolerant of people who weren't doing what I felt was a good job. Sometimes I was unable to control that anger. I didn't like to be questioned and I didn't like to be challenged. Sometimes my anger would flare up like a gasoline fire, then be gone as quickly as it had come. I could not control it, and could not live with its aftermath. I was not completely sure where it came from inside me. Many surgeons I have known have had this tendency to deal with difficult situations with anger. Had I unintentionally adopted this personality? Was it just impatience with laziness or incompetence? Was it a deeply felt, long-term anger over the deterioration of my culture that spilled into other areas of my life? I did not know. I knew that I still had many deficiencies when it came to my bedside manner and my "surgical personality." I was not the warmest person in the world because I didn't let people get too close to me. I wanted to be a better doctor, and I looked to the Navajo tradition of healing for answers.

From a Navajo standpoint, illness can be caused by an imbalance or lack of harmony in any area of a patient's life. I began to realize that *everything* a patient encounters has an impact on her. If illness could be caused by a lack of harmony, could not the same be true for wellness and the ability to heal? It made sense that if the healing environment was more "harmonious," a patient might return to wellness faster.

Why is it that some doctors do an operation right but their patients die? I asked. *Why do some procedures go so seriously wrong?* It had to do with other things besides the procedures and instruments, besides the preconditions of patients. It had to do with stress, fear, and the problems of the surgery.

After what happened with Evelyn, it became clearer to me why there were so many difficulties. I had operated on a patient I hardly knew, stepping in for another surgeon (something we all try to avoid) at the last minute, assuming that all would be well. I had not developed any bond of trust or acceptance in advance. During her operation, her body had been anything but cooperative, and I cringed when I thought of how either Evelyn or her spirit may have listened as I ranted during the surgery. She had no doubt sensed my own discomfort, fatigue, frustration, and anger. And the nurses had argued with each other. Even when patients are anesthetized, there is some evidence that they hear what goes on during surgery and respond to what is happening. Some surgeons or anesthesiologists will play music while operating. This is in part for their own enjoyment, but it also must soothe the patient.

Was the stroke Evelyn's body's response to the disharmony that had prevailed during her surgery? I would never know for sure. But I had been taught a powerful lesson, and I promised myself I would become more sensitive, work on my temper, and never let such conditions interfere with a patient's treatment again, if I could help it. I had to try harder to make sure that patients felt comfortable. Perhaps I could set up my practice so that the occasions for frustration and anger would be rare. Or maybe, by working closer with nurses, staff, and other doctors, by trying to prevent problems before they arose, I could create greater harmony in my own surgical world, which could make things better for everyone on the team.

Before a surgeon proceeds with an operation, it is important that she obtain the patient's trust and acceptance, as is making sure that the patient wants to have the surgery done, that the doctor is not just talking them into it. They must understand the procedure that will be performed on them. And during the procedure, there should be a sense of *hózhǫ́* and beauty in the OR. My spirit and the patient's spirit can work together to make the surgery successful, I thought. They will encourage a positive outcome.

In the Navajo world traditional healers are expected to lead by example. They teach their patients to Walk in Beauty in part by Walking in Beauty themselves. There is no correlate for this practice in Western medicine. Physicians work and live under conditions of great stress, and there is little cultural expectation that they will take care of themselves or set an example for their patients. In a Western health care system the different components are under no obligation to work smoothly together. Because of this the results are widely variable; some relationships are cordial, but others can be antagonistic, if not downright hostile. If all the members of my team worked together harmoniously and in concert, I thought, and if we tried to gain the trust, respect, and understanding of the patient, we could create better surgical outcomes. We ourselves would be happier and less stressed as well.

I looked at every part of our hospital to see if we could do a better job of making our patients relaxed and comfortable. There were factors that could make all the difference in the world: at GIMC, many of the nurses were Navajo or from other tribes, as were many of the maintenance and secretarial staff. At night, when almost everyone else had gone home, it made the patients feel safe to have Navajo speakers caring for them.

Similarly, early on, I saw the benefits of a doctor speaking to patients in their own language. Ruby Billy and Rosemary Ramone, two of our surgical nurses, quietly and clearly spoke to elderly female patients about the surgery or treatment they needed in their native tongue. The difference was striking: these women's facial expressions were invariably calmer and more trusting.

A ten-year-old girl with a hernia was brought into the OR for an operation. She had a beautiful, innocent face, but fear was clearly etched in her eyes. Valden would make her unconscious by giving her a cocktail of anesthetic gases that had been designed specifically for her weight and age. Dressed in the blue scrubs over his old cowboy boots, Valden whispered reassuring Navajo words into her ear as she fell asleep: *"Ił wosh shiyázh."* ("Go to sleep, little one"). The fear in her face dissipated.

Soon I began using bits of Navajo with my own patients. I began to say, *"Ni bid neezgai'ish?"* ("Does your stomach hurt?") I told them in their own language I would need to operate on them: *"Ni tl'izh ndeeshgizh"* ("We're going to operate on your gallbladder"). At the end of every examination I would ask *"Nabídiłkid?"* ("Do you have any questions?") The faces of the older people would relax when the person who would perform their procedures spoke to them in their own language.

▲▲▲▲

During this time I also adjusted to the patients' levels of comfort about touching. I would touch my patients, as Dr. Lujan does, only when necessary and always in an extremely respectful fashion. Remembering my own illness at

Stanford, I also adjusted the way I viewed patients. I looked at them as if they were all members of my extended family, which in a sense they were. We were all *Diné*—the People.

Once in a while, a medicine man would come into the hospital and perform a ceremony right at a patient's bedside. I watched this in awe. Only a few major hospitals permitted such practices. The patients immediately responded positively to the visit of a *hataałii*, or medicine man. It was clear that they *believed* he would heal them. Then these patients' conditions would often improve. The evidence was anecdotal, to be sure, but finding funding for a double-blind clinical study of the phenomenon would be hard to come by—not to mention the fact that the patients and medicine men wouldn't agree to participate. I asked other doctors at GIMC for their impressions, and they concurred: patients treated by *hataałii* had better outcomes. To accommodate these traditional ceremonies, some IHS clinics and hospitals (such as ACL, Chinle, and Shiprock) had built *kivas* or holy ceremonial rooms right onto the hospital facilities. The National Institutes of Mental Health had even financed the training of medicine men in *Dinétah*, to address the problem of their declining numbers. Fewer younger men were choosing to follow in the footsteps of their elders and learn the complicated ceremonies, sand paintings, and songs of our people. The NIMH had recognized the importance of this tradition and allocated funding to preserve it.

I had to wonder: If Evelyn Bitsui had had a singer at her side before surgery, if that person had given her the confidence and certainty that harmony would be restored in her life, would she have suffered a stroke?

Seeing how well patients reacted to the presence of a traditional healer made me want to become more of a healer myself. But I had little idea how to go about it. Such a pursuit was not something one dabbled in—it was a life work. It would be impossible for me to learn all the songs and ceremonies of a medicine man in one lifetime. But maybe somehow my practice could incorporate some elements of Navajo beliefs and philosophies and a respect for our ways. This would be a very strong kind of medicine, I thought, mixing together the best of both worlds.

Chapter Five

▲▲▲▲

REZ DOGS
AND CROW DREAMS

*Dreams gather quickly
like Spring crows,
and they scatter.*

—SIMON ORTIZ,
"Returned from California"[5]

I was on morning rounds in the intensive care unit. The smell of coffee, cooling in our cups, mixed with the smell of freshly cleaned linens. A computer screen, divided into bright purple and green lines, traced the activities of the patients' hearts, a stack of their charts lay on the counter.

With my fellow surgeon Susan Stuart and a specialist in internal medicine, Terry Sloan, I waited for everyone else to arrive. As people filed in, several nurses chatted by the doorway. An old audiotape was playing, and music poured through the serious air like honey. Then someone turned down the music, and we began to make our rounds, going over the histories of each patient. (All names of patients have been changed to protect confidentiality.)

Bed 66: Slim, Ray, a 38-year-old male with early cirrhosis and active hepatitis,

fevers, a high white count, and pancreatitis. He
was described as a "binge-type drinker who spends
his weekends intoxicated."

Bed 65: Thompson, Robert, a 51-year-old male
with severe cirrhosis, ulcers, and internal
bleeding. Needs an esophagogastroduodenoscopy,
or "scope," to locate the source of bleeding in his
intestinal tract.

Bed 67: Redhouse, Betty, a 29-year-old woman
with a bleeding ulcer, heart condition, and severe
liver damage. In the hospital because of a beating
that was believed to have been the result of a
domestic violence incident. She has lacerations
and cuts to the head and neck, as well as a long
knife wound to the abdomen.

Bed 64: Antonio, Henry, a 38-year-old man with
massive trauma to the neck, mild wheezing,
mild hypoxia, severely lacerated tongue, a
lumbar fracture, and multiple fractures in the
left ankle.

As the physicians talked, this last patient's story began to
unfold. Henry Antonio had been jailed the previous night
for drunk and disorderly behavior and had tried to hang
himself in his jail cell. He suffered back and ankle injuries
when he fell. It was believed he had a seizure after the
hanging attempt. That was when he bit off part of his
tongue.

Listening to the doctors describe these patients in detail
on that late winter morning, the fractured and unharmo-
nious parts of our community came into focus, as did one
of its chief causes. These patient cases and many of those
that followed on that round had a common denominator:

alcohol. Much of what I was dealing with medically in the intensive care unit was either directly related to or a side effect of alcohol. Daily, again and again, I found myself forced to consider this toxic substance and the serious damage it was doing to people.

I was not naive about alcohol. In some ways drugs are not unknown to Native cultures, which traditionally used some form of hallucinogenic or mind-altering substance as a part of their religious practices. Yet alcohol is different. It has a devastating, dramatic, and negative effect. Very early on in our history, alcohol was outlawed on reservations, possibly for paternalistic reasons, but bars and liquor stores always spring up nearby.

The lives of the patients at GIMC were scarred by the disease of alcoholism. Making rounds in the intensive care unit made it obvious: this was an epidemic.

Gallup has about fifty bars to serve fifty thousand people, and arrests for driving intoxicated exceed ten thousand a year. The opening of several new government alcohol treatment programs and the city of Gallup's ban on drive-up liquor sales improved the situation somewhat, but the problem did not go away. The incidence of fetal alcohol syndrome, a condition caused by mothers drinking during pregnancy, is the highest in the country among Native people. Through its pervasiveness and its availability, alcohol has touched the lives of Navajos on many levels.

Alcohol has been called one of the "lubricants of domination," given to non-Europeans by Europeans.[6] Every day I saw cirrhosis, hepatitis, ulcers, internal bleeding, pancreatitis, domestic violence–related injuries—all pathologies that could be associated with the excessive or habitual ingestion of alcohol. We bandaged them up, dried them out, and sent them on their way, but many times they'd be back.

Even after I had been in Gallup only a short while I had already encountered a vast number of patients whose lives were trapped and tangled in alcohol-related problems.

One day as I was operating at GIMC with Greg Stephens and one of our anesthesiologists, Daryl Smith, both of whom were black, I overheard their conversation about people they'd grown up with. They cited the well-known tragedy about young black men in this country: That many of their male childhood friends have been killed or were in jail. They named names, ticking them off on their fingers, and remembered the casualties. Suddenly it dawned on me: many of the children I grew up with on the reservation were no longer alive either—but nobody ever really talked about the high number of teenage Indian casualties: Rena Craig, Ernie Henry, Adrian Tenequer, Alfred Chavez, the Howard brothers, Rickey Estevan, Elmer Morgan, Leroy Etcitty, Roger Etcitty. Dead not from guns and drugs but from alcohol, suicide, and automobiles—our own lethal combination. I recalled their faces, one by one, and my spirit ached with their loss.

The leading cause of death among Navajos isn't liver disease or pancreatitis—it is motor vehicle accidents. The rate is three times higher for men than for women; the highest percentage of all is for men in the 25-to-34 age range. Indian Health Service statistics estimate that 60 percent of those accidents are alcohol related, and the numbers are rising.

Besides accidents, other alcohol-related incidents were also common. Everett Nelson, a teenager, was brought in with long tears and crisscross rips in his body from knife wounds. He said his brother and he had gotten in a fight, but his tattoos and clothing told a different story. Gangs on the reservation had been increasing for a decade or so and I was seeing the result.

Young Navajo men like Everett, not yet seventeen, would come in with gunshot or stab wounds. There were even a gang-related fatality in Shiprock: a fourteen-year-old

Navajo boy named Shoshonnie Francisco. The gang culture was yet one more outside influence—this time of imported violence and territoriality—that threatened Navajo culture. No one knows for sure how it first infiltrated the far-flung sheep camps and washes of the rez, but it did. Before long Navajo schoolchildren were wearing the symbols and colors of the Bloods and Crips of the West Coast gangs. Soon afterward they began to show up in GIMC, like Everett, and were some of my most seriously injured patients. Navajo communities have become increasingly alarmed by this trend. The elders say that it is a result of the fact that parents have not taught their children the traditional ways. Without the teachings of Walking in Beauty, these children attempted to create their own tribe, but with devastating effects. The blueprint for tribal lifeways had not been handed down to them. Alcohol only made the violence and gang-related crime worse. Usually it took place when they were drunk.

Standing in the intensive care unit that morning and many other mornings in the years that followed, surrounded by patients whose illnesses could all be traced to the abuse of alcohol, I realized that in my profession as a surgeon, I would see the saddest side of this disease—the casualties. I would treat their sick livers and stomachs, and I would treat their bleeding bodies. But there would be little I could do about their souls, the captives of a cruel substance that would probably never let them go. Almost every Navajo family had a member with an alcohol problem.

In my own family that person was my father. Soon after I arrived in Gallup and began practicing surgery at GIMC, my medical work and my personal life came together in a tragic intersection.

My father's story showed me in a personal way how alcohol is destroying our community. When I got back to Dine-tah, I saw his alcoholism differently than I had before I left. Before, I had seen it as a problem in our family, but now I also saw it as a disease, in a clinical fashion. Because of him I was able to look at my patients as individuals, each with their own particular story and paths to this illness. Our historic grief had led to a collectively experienced plague; my father was the window through which I could see it.

Robert Cupp, my father, was by any culture's standards an extraordinary man. He had a gift for speaking to animals. Almost everywhere we went, on the reservation or off, he knew the dogs, and they recognized him and came running. Rez dogs. Chocolate and black-splotched or the color of coyote and mesa and riverbed mud. One blue eye, one brown, or two piercing green. They are everywhere on the reservation, used to watch the sheep or guard the hogan, and when you arrive they appear magically, just like those annoying friends who materialize at mealtime. My father knew them. Crows also seemed to gather in groups or come and stand on a fencepost whenever my father was around. Sometimes I'd turn a corner and find my father standing deep in a philosophical discussion with a crow.

In the Navajo world, where everything is connected, talking to animals or acknowledging their presence is not as unusual as it is in other places. In addition to fluent crow and rez dog, my dad sometimes seemed to know the dialects of deer, elk, and even trout—he could easily decipher their language of leaps and cautious lingering in the pools made by rocky eddies. He taught his daughters how to hunt, how to look at a certain set of tracks and determine instantly what type of animal it was from its size, and how long ago it had passed. My two sisters became accomplished hunters. I would usually go along but sit on a rock and read. He also taught us camping and boating and showed us how to hand tie fishing flies.

But perhaps the most important thing about my father was

that he taught us the simplest things—Navajo things—like how to just sit and be quiet, to blend in and watch, or to move so silently we'd become a part of the forest. My father taught us how to live the concepts of our culture, especially the importance of communicating with the natural world.

For most Native people the animals and environment have a spirit and life of their own that is respected and protected. Part of the Beauty Way ceremony teaches us that humans should live in harmony with the animal world and the natural world—the earth, plants, water, air, everything that surrounds us. Navajo chantways are beautiful in their descriptions of the world we live in. For example, the Mountain Chantway has passages that capture the power and glory of nature:

> *The voice that beautifies the land!*
> *The voice above*
> *The voice of the thunder*
> *Within the dark cloud,*
> *Again and again it sounds,*
> *The voice that beautifies the land!*
> *The voice of the grasshopper*
> *Among the plants,*
> *Again and again it sounds,*
> *The voice that beautifies the land!*[7]

My father taught us that before a hunt traditionally raised Navajos sang sacred songs. He also taught us that part of the meat must be given away, and that nothing should be wasted.

Our family honored that tradition by providing meat for my father's grandparents and other elder relatives, and by wasting nothing. We could not even leave any meat on the ribs we ate.

In their childhoods both my father and my grandmother had been punished for speaking Navajo in school. White educators believed that, in order to be successful, Navajos would have to forget their language and culture and adopt American ways. They were warned that if they taught their children to speak Navajo, the children would have a harder time learning in school, and would therefore be at a disadvantage.

A racist attitude existed. Navajo children were told that their culture and lifeways were inferior, and they were made to feel they could never be as good as white people. This pressure to assimilate, along with the physical, social, psychological, and economic destruction of the tribes following the Indian wars of the 1800s, the poverty due to poor grazing lands and forced stock reduction, and the lack of available jobs all combined to bring the Navajo people to their knees. The physical genocide of the 1800s, followed by the cultural genocide of the 1900s, left behind a tribe whose roots and foundation were shattered.

My father suffered terribly from these events and conditions. He had been a straight-A student and was sent away to one of the best prep schools in the state. He wanted to be like the rich white children who surrounded him there, but the differences were too apparent. My father resented the limitations that being Navajo presented in the 1940s and 1950s. He went to the University of New Mexico, majoring in premed and Latin. It was there that he met my mother.

"She looked so angelic," he often said about their first encounter. To the Navajo boy who was taught to feel shame about the color of his skin, she must have. My mother has blond hair and blue eyes, and she probably represented everything that he felt he was not. When they married, my dad left college and went to White Horse Lake to run the trading post, leaving behind his academic dreams. Not long afterward he began to hate himself for being unable to fit into the white world and for not fulfilling his dreams. He escaped his grief with alcohol and would disappear for days, sometimes weeks. I remember the empty seat at the dinner table when he was gone. At those times his absence was a presence. We'd walk around the house, acutely aware of all the places he wasn't—his workshop, the yard, his favorite chair in the living room.

Once, in the middle of the night I was lying with my sisters in the backseat of the car in my pajamas. It was like so many other nights, that night, but somehow it has stayed intact in my memory, almost like a film.

Karen, Robyn, and I waited amid a heap of blankets and pillows while my mother searched for my dad in the bars on Gallup's main strip. We'd already been by the police stations in both Gallup and Crownpoint. Our last stop was the Gallup morgue, where an unidentified Indian man lay dead. Mom had heard about it from a man in one of the bars and didn't want to explain it to us. But we knew where we were, and we knew why we were there. Karen, Robyn, and I huddled together in our blankets while she went in to see if the face beneath the white sheet was his. It wasn't, but when she came out, she looked stark white and shaken.

After I went away to college, my father cut way back on his binges. But always, whenever he was gone, there was uncertainty and fear. I would wonder if he was okay, if he'd been arrested, or if he lay hurt somewhere, the victim of an accident, or if someone else had been injured as well. In our house, whenever the phone rang and Dad was away, we would exchange heavy glances. Such calls often brought bad news.

My father really was two people. One was the man who took pride in everything we did. He never missed a single one of Karen's basketball games. He played for hours with Robyn's baby son, B.J., and read *Parents* magazine.

The other man had black fire streaming through his veins,

his life dreams scattered like frightened crows. Alcohol had erased these dreams. It had also enslaved him, as it had so many patients I saw. When I came into work and saw so many cases involving the deterioration of the body through alcohol, I would remind myself that each one had a story, each one a reason why.

Two or three generations of our tribe had been taught to feel shame about our culture, and parents had often not taught their children traditional Navajo beliefs—the very thing that would have shown them how to live, the very thing that could keep them strong.

▲▲▲▲

Today the tire marks have faded, where they left the highway on Interstate 40 near mile marker 47. I saw them all winter in 1993, two years after I came home to practice medicine. A pair of bright black parallel lines veered off the pavement to the right. The site was located between my house in Gallup and my parents' house near Grants, so I had no choice but to drive by it again and again as I came to visit my family. One day I noticed that I could no longer see the tracks, but it didn't matter, I'd memorized them. It was the place where my father's car had rolled four times before smashing into an iron rail.

Each time I saw that place I whispered, *"Ayóó ninshné."* I love you, Dad.

My father is buried in a beautiful, manicured cemetery in Albuquerque. But that is not where he is. I have been in that cemetery many times; I do not feel his presence. In fact, I often forget that he is there at all. Not so at mile marker 47. To the east is Mount Taylor, our beautiful, sacred Tsoodzil. It seems ironic that nearby, also, was the Top of the World, his favorite bar, at the town of Continental Divide.

It is as though this place were chosen for him.

Mile marker 47. My father's spirit pulled me each time I passed it. It was as though he cast out with his fly-fishing rod there, and it hooked my soul.

▲▲▲▲

Chapter Six

CEREMONY MEDICINE

*There are medicines for lightning. There are
medicines for bear wounds and the same for
snakes. There are medicines for evil done by
water. There are medicines against all those
who do harm. With our Life Way medicines,
people get well. A person who is broken
all over, even he can survive with these
medicines. We have songs for preparing the
medicines . . . that's how we pray to be cured!
That is how people get well.*

—GEORGE BLUEEYES,
Navajo medicine man

There is no word for *cancer* in the Navajo
language.

In the beginning of my tenure at GIMC I described it to my patients as a "bad sickness" that
grows inside and will spread if not treated. Soon I
tried to use phrases I had heard Roy Smith use:
'ats'íís naałdzid (which translates loosely as "a sore
that does not heal") or *natzee* ("something that
rots"). By naming it in Navajo, Roy had made it
into a force, a natural element, something the pa-

tients could understand the way they understood lightning, rain, snow, and the seasons.

But somehow, when I said the same words, they were lacking. Each time I encountered a patient who needed to be referred to an oncologist, I struggled with the dilemma. They could not really comprehend this ailment, which defied all logic and natural reasoning. They seemed to suspect that this "bad sickness" that could not be seen was an invention of the doctors.

My patients responded to the news that they had the "bad sickness" in all sorts of different ways. There are strong superstitions about cancer among Navajos who know of it, fears and beliefs that were almost as hard to deal with as the cancer itself.

Rose Becenti, from Naschitti, was an older woman who had advanced cancer of the rectum. When I explained her condition to her, and the radical and disturbing surgery she needed, she didn't believe me. She knew what was wrong with her. "I was struck by lightning, long, long time ago," she told me. A medicine man had given her a drink to cure her of the lightning sickness, she said, and she hadn't drunk all of it. She simply needed to get the rest of the lightning out of her, she said. She was going back to visit him. She left the hospital, and I never saw her again.

I treated patients whose families could not believe the disease was not contagious. One afternoon a week before Christmas, I found myself face-to-face with a beautiful woman, my own age and height, with large, intelligent eyes. She was full-blooded Navajo, with high, rounded cheeks and long, thick, straight hair fixed in a tight blue-black braid.

Like me, Carolyn Yazzie had been away to college, and she now held a professional job in a government office in Windowrock, the capital of the Navajo Nation. She seemed confident and strong and introduced herself to me in Navajo by her clans. "I was born into the *Bįįh Din'e'é* or 'deer people,'

and born 'for' [her father's side] the *To'áháni* or 'near to water' clan," she said. I could not help but feel a kinship with
her. I think she felt the same way toward me.

We talked about the weather—the high winds we'd been
having, and the snow we should have been having but
weren't—and then she told me a little about her parents and
Lukaichukai, the place where she grew up on the reservation.
Then finally, with hesitation, she began to tell me her story. I
realized she was terrified.

She looked out the window for a minute. Then she blurted
out, "My sister won't eat my fry bread. Nobody will. It just
sits on the table and gets hard." She looked at me for a second, hoping I'd understand. "Only flies go near it."

Ever since she had been to the clinic at Fort Defiance
and found out about the lump in her breast, people in her
life had been avoiding her. For weeks, not only would they
not touch her food, they wouldn't touch her. At her office
some of the secretaries would leave the room when she entered, or move to the side whenever she passed, as though
she had the kind of repellent power of a magnet. Even her
own husband and children, she said, swayed from her
touch.

I examined her breast, moving out from the nipple in cir-
cular motions, until I found it—a hard center with thickened
breast tissue around it. Her tumor.

Even though it was almost Christmas and the biopsy could
probably wait until after the holidays, I scheduled one for her
the following week. I knew that if her tumor turned out to be
malignant, it would most likely be a stage-one tumor. While
there are no promises with cancer, stage one is usually cur-
able. But it could also spread up into the lymph nodes below
her arm; and through her lymphatic system, it could be mi-
grating to other parts of her body.

Carolyn's story had scared me. Since then, I'd found myself almost unconsciously checking my own breasts in the

shower or while getting dressed, for the hard pebblelike sign of the disease that claims so many women's lives.

Anyone who has ever had cancer or lost a relative or friend to it knows how the disease ransacks the body. The explosion of abnormal cells can cause the organs to fail one by one, eventually leading to death. Even today, with all our technology and millions of dollars of research funds, we do not know nearly enough about why it happens or how to stop it. In the broader society, superstitions and folklore still surround it. Even though cancer is associated with definite causes such as smoking and hereditary factors, other theories about what can cause it range from stress and injury to diet.

Among Navajos, I soon learned, cancer is even further mythologized. Some believe that cancer, like certain other illnesses, is caused by an evil action or a bad deed of the person who falls sick. Many do not understand that it cannot be virally transmitted from person to person, like chicken pox or the measles—other white man's illnesses.

Some of the other doctors in Gallup told me sad stories about their cancer patients. These patients might turn up at other, faraway clinics, sometimes on the other side of the reservation. Their families would drop them off there, leaving the relative with cancer behind, returning three or even four hundred miles to their homes. What these families were basically saying to health care workers was "Take this person"—a very unusual thing for Navajo people to do, who tend to be zealously loyal to their families. A few days after I performed the biopsy, Carolyn's results came back. The lump was breast cancer. Maybe my own fears of the disease caused me to speak bluntly to Carolyn, like a *bilagáana*.

"I think you should have this surgery soon," I told her in one of the small examining rooms at GIMC. I then tried to explain it carefully, in a Navajo way, so that she could understand that it was not something she had caused, and that it probably could not be stopped without an operation. I then explained that we would need to remove the breast tissue around the lump (a lumpectomy) and some of her lymph nodes in her axilla (an axillary dissection).

In the best of all possible worlds, I'd thought, surgery, chemo/radiation, and a traditional ceremony or "sing" would all be available to cancer patients. It is very hard to heal a person who does not believe they will get well, or a person who does not want to. Most doctors will agree that such patients fare very poorly. A sing by a *hataałii* gives Navajo patients a dimension to their cure that is often crucial to their survival. By this time, after watching my own patients deal with cancer in different ways, I had come to believe strongly that such treatment would increase the remission rate of Navajo cancer patients. These patients prepared themselves mentally and spiritually to fight their disease, a very Navajo concept. I wanted to tell Carolyn to arrange a sing for herself, but I didn't know quite how to broach the subject.

Although she had gone to college, Carolyn and her family were traditional Navajos and lived a rural life. I told her she needed a lumpectomy and might need to follow that up with chemotherapy and radiation, with referral to an oncologist. Then I finally suggested it. "If you'd like," I said, "we can wait until you see a medicine man first. But I don't want you to wait too long."

Carolyn looked at me for a moment without speaking, then looked away. Silence filled the room like a single, long, inconclusive sentence. Then she turned to me and said she wasn't sure. A medicine man had visited her grandfather the previous year—she would see about finding him. But she also told me she didn't know if she wanted the surgery. "I'd like some time to think about it," she said.

I looked into her eyes, something Navajos don't usually do. She was a woman so much like myself, who had been to college, who had some understanding of the gravity of what she was saying. Letting the cancer go could be a terrible mistake. "Don't think too long," I said.

A few weeks went by with no word from her. I wanted to call, but I also wanted to give her time to think. Then one morning one of the OR nurses told me that a young woman was having a sing that weekend. It was Yeibechei (pronounced yāy bi-chāy), and many people were going.

Could it be Carolyn Yazzie? I wondered. I had not been to a Yeibechei, the last night of a Night Chant ceremony, in many years, since I was a child. A Night Chant is a ceremony held in the dead of winter for a sick person. Its purpose is to restore that person's harmony. Many of the Navajo gods, like Talking God (Haashch'ééłtii), appear. The families hire dancers to perform. Medicine men come and make sand paintings and offer special prayers. The Night Chant is nine nights long, and the last night, the most spectacular and important night, is the Yeibechei.

Suddenly I was filled with a desire to go to the Yeibechei that night. Entrenched as I was in Western medicine and my surgical practice, I wanted to see the *Diné* healing medicine again. I wanted to smell the Yeibechei and see the people gathered in the winter dark.

I asked where it would be held. A nurse from my clan— we'd discovered it during an appendectomy one day—said I could join them if I wanted. I planned to follow them out in my car, so I could leave the ceremony earlier if I wanted. The Yeibechei could last all night, but I wasn't sure I could, having been on call the previous night. But I wanted to see Carolyn Yazzie wrapped in blankets before a hogan filled with sand paintings made to cure her. I left a message at her house asking her to call, but at three-thirty I still had no word.

When I got home, I flipped on the television, looking for a distraction as I prepared dinner for my grandmother and myself.

Conroy Chino, Channel Four's news anchor, an Indian from Acoma Pueblo, called for a "no burn" night. In Albuquerque on windless nights the smoke from fires gets trapped in the basin of the Rio Grande Valley. On a "no burn" night no one would be able to warm themselves by fireside. But just a few hours later, deep in Dinetah, I stood among five huge piñon fires burning furiously, stoked with pieces of wood so huge that each could be an entire tree trunk. The flames shot into the dark sky and sent up plumes of orange sparks that twirled overhead, as if to conspire with the ceiling of bright white stars. A tingling of anticipation and excitement filled the air. It was a traditional winter ceremony: a Yeibechei.

In the center of the winter night was a hogan, surrounded by a cluster of parked pickup trucks. Before the hogan stood a chair covered with Pendleton and hand-woven Navajo blankets. In the chair sat a girl.

She was tall. You could tell by the length of her legs, swathed in blankets, protruding in front of her. She was lovely; around her head was tied a red sash. She was not Carolyn.

I did not know this young woman or her family, but she was clearly sick. That was why she was sitting wrapped in blankets on this cold January night in front of the hogan, expressionless. She was there to be cured.

The nurses, whom I had followed for many miles in my car from Gallup to arrive there, were friends of the girl's family, as was everyone crowding around the fires before the hogan for warmth. Grandmothers sat in folding lawn chairs, wrapped in blankets, unmoving. Men and women stamped their feet to stay warm, and children held on to their hands or played quietly beside them. Teenagers huddled in small groups around the periphery. A tiny concession stand, set up in the back of somebody's pickup truck, dispensed fry bread, boiled coffee, tea, and mutton sandwiches wrapped in oily paper towels. Some of the men were wearing cowboy hats; others' caps bore the names of various sports teams.

On this night everyone had come together for one reason: Talking God would dance in the firelight, beneath the thick silver belt of the Milky Way, to cure this girl. The songs of the Night Chant tell of the beauty of the Navajo universe:

> *House made of dawn*
> *House made of evening light*
> *House made of the dark cloud*
> *Dark cloud is at the house's door,*
> *The trail out of it is dark cloud*
> *The zigzag lightning stands high upon it*
> *Happily may I walk*
> *Happily with abundant showers, may I walk*
> *Happily with abundant plants, may I walk*
> *Happily, on the trail of pollen, may I walk.*
> *Happily may I walk.*
> *May it be beautiful before me.*
> *May it be beautiful behind me.*
> *May it be beautiful below me.*
> *May it be beautiful above me*
> *May it be beautiful all around me.*
>
> *In beauty it is finished.*

The Yeibechei has to be held on a winter night, "when the snakes are sleeping and before the thunder comes." As I scanned the sea of faces, I saw a couple of *bilagáanas* in the crowd. Maybe they were the girl's schoolteachers or coaches. I recognized a few faces—Navajos; they'd come by way of a word-of-mouth invitation only. There is no formal, written announcement of a Yeibechei. The only way to know about it is to hear of it from a friend, or a friend of a friend, or a family member. To get there means driving over dirt roads that forked off dirt roads in the heart of the rez, following a cavalcade of pickups that split the deep darkness of the mesas with the twin beams of their headlights.

Before the ceremony the girl may have gone, as many of my traditional patients did, to see a crystal gazer or hand trembler. That person would be an older man or woman, who uses a crystal and what seems to be a sensitivity to magnetism, electricity, or other forces in the human body. He or she would diagnose her and recommend a particular type of ceremony, such as this Night Chant.

It is said that everyone who attends a Night Chant benefits from the ceremony's healing power. Perhaps that explained, in part, the size of the crowd assembled here—they would stay all night long, outside, in the dead of winter. But they were also there because it was what they should do: be there on this night.

As I stood in the freezing winter air, the backs of my legs were seared by the heat of the bonfire flames, while the rest of me grew cold, facing the chill. A medicine man and another man were conferring about their patient, standing on either side of the girl in the chair before the hogan. A lot of activity was going on inside the hogan, but only family members would be allowed to enter that sanctuary tonight. For the past few days sand paintings had been made at dawn there and destroyed by twilight. Prayer sticks, mutton sandwiches, and bowls of chili had been prepared to feed the many people who would come for the ceremony.

A woman came out and wrapped an extra blanket around the girl and placed a basket with corn pollen in her lap. The yellow light from inside the hogan glowed through the doorway like the rectangular mouth of a jack-o'-lantern. Then someone pulled the woven-rug door closed. Beyond the makeshift parking lot, shapes emerged from the dark emptiness. It was the dancers.

At first there were only three, and they approached slowly. They were nearly naked, wearing only small skirts of wool and moccasins, their bodies painted white with ash. The first was Hashch'eelti'i, Talking God, whose face was a mask of painted buckskin and eagle feathers. He danced toward the girl with a bouncing movement, spruce branches wreathing his neck. Behind him was Water Sprinkler, a clown, and behind him, third and last in the group, a figure completely hunched over, like an arthritic old man. It was Yaaskidi, the hunchback, whose wooden cane spoked into three branches at the bottom, like a claw. Their feet stamped in unison. They shook the rattles in their right hands. Then Talking God let loose a series of cries that echoed four times in the cold air. Together they began to chant a song that belonged to the night.

The song was repetitive and rhythmic, causing a rush of memories inside me. The singing was all in the lower vocal register, filled with solemnity and magic. The Night Chant, like all our ceremonies, is believed to be a gift from the *yei,* or ancient holy people, all of whom had come to visit the *Diné* during this ceremony. (Note: Although some of the names of the *Diné* holy people have been translated as "God," such as "Talking God," they are more correctly referred to as holy beings. The concept of the creator in *Diné* belief is complex, but it includes the concept of "Sa'a Naaghai Bik'e Hozho": a life force that creates all things, connects all things, and is within all things; the creator is the universe, and the universe has a consciousness of which we are all part.)

The sick girl got up from her chair and pulled the blankets around her tightly. She walked over to the three *yei* dancers and with a wandlike wave of her arm, sprinkled corn pollen onto each of them. Then she went back and sat down in the chair.

The dancers shook their rattles in sweeping gestures toward the earth and went back to the place where they had come from. Their brightness closed back into the dark envelope of the mesa.

I pulled my coat around me for warmth and watched my

breath condense in the cold air like a tiny cloud. A short while later the process was repeated, but with different dancers. Talking God was still there, but he was accompanied by eight others. Next came a group of sixteen, in pairs of women and men. All wore the masks that transformed them into Navajo holy people. All were wreathed in pine branches and carried rattles. Their moccasined feet shuffled in rhythmic unison as they chanted before the girl, who sprinkled each one with corn pollen. Sometimes Talking God was stalked by a clown who mocked him. Instead of eagle feathers, he had turkey feathers around his head, and his movements were exaggerated imitations of Talking God.

All the people were there to help the girl get well—and she must be aware of the power of their collected presence around her, I thought. She could feel, see, and smell the Yeibechei medicine. It was hypnotic: the repetitive chants, the smell, swirl, and string of woodsmoke, the rattles and rhythms of the drums, the appearance and disappearance of the groups of dancers. In spite of my medical training, I knew that being surrounded by one's family and greater community for nine days, and seeing dancing gods smudged with gray ash, bringing healing chants from the dark mesa beyond the bonfires, would have a very positive effect on her condition, whatever it may be. Ceremonies are magical and powerful things. A spiritual intensity and an energy surrounds the healing ceremony that is almost completely absent in Western medicine. Centrally, however, the purpose of the ceremony is to help the patient return to a way of thinking and living in harmony and balance, which helps guide the patient's body back to health. While at Stanford I had yearned for something like it for my non-Indian patients there, who went through their operations alone or nearly alone. Their minds and spirits were often not prepared for surgery and could not assist in healing them, nor did their families and communities come together for the purpose of helping them heal. I wondered if other people whose ancestors had been part of tribes centuries ago yearned for tribal identity. In the roar of the Yeibechei fires, beneath the starry sky, I felt how lucky I was to be a part of my tribe. Even though the Night Chant hadn't been for Carolyn Yazzie, I was glad I had come.

I had been attending more traditional events since I came back to *Dinétah*. Earlier that winter, Eunice Jamon, a Zuni Indian who was one of our OR scrub nurses, had invited me to a night of dances called the Shalako. As I was getting ready to go, Grandma gave me a hard time.

"Oh, you're going to freeze out there—and there will be nothing to see."

"That's not true, Grandma. We'll see the Shalako."

"They're always having dancing over there," she said. Once when we were driving by Zuni and I pointed out their holy mountain, she had said: "If you spit in Zuni it hits something holy."

After I came home from the Yeibechei I could smell the smoke and the night on my coat and in my hair, and I suddenly remembered vividly all those feast days of my childhood. Our family—especially Dad—had always loved the Zuni pueblos and for many years we went to their ceremonies and feast days. He especially loved to take us to Laguna for the throw-outs—feasts where the Laguna people actually throw gifts off their roofs to visitors. Most of the time these were groceries or practical items, but sometimes they were expensive pottery. And sometimes an expectant crowd had nothing but water showered on them!

Shush and Bouncer seemed excited to smell the wood-smoke smell clinging to me. Since I had been home, I had not experienced this kind of magic and I felt different because of it. I had experienced my tribe's medicine again. It had been a long time and I knew that that Night Chant had helped "cure" me as well.

But I was still worried: The medicine had not been for Carolyn. I was faced with a dilemma. I wanted to call her up

and say "Carolyn, how are you? Have you come to any decisions about the surgery?"

But that would violate traditional Navajo boundaries of
what was appropriate. It is considered impolite and an invasion of privacy to ask too many questions of a person. I
would soon be asking the risk management office of GIMC
to send her an official letter, informing her of her condition
in writing and urging her to seek treatment. This was mainly
a maneuver designed to protect the hospital legally. I fought
off a desire to drive up toward Windowrock and speak to her.
Finally, days later, just as I was finishing up an examination
of another patient, she called me.

"Carolyn," I said. "I have been waiting to hear from you."

"My sister told me that this—cancer—is my fault," she
said.

I could see that she was looking at her illness in a very
natural way for a Navajo. She was looking for its cause. In a
harmonious world every effect has a cause.

"You didn't do anything," I told her. To her family, Carolyn's cancer meant she might have done something evil, and
the evil had then reappeared in her own body. But Carolyn
could not think of what she had done. She'd stayed up late
nights combing over her life, trying to remember.

Even though she knew about genetics, environmental haz-
ards, and so forth, she was dwelling on her own actions: what
in her life lacked beauty? It was difficult for me to explain to
her that people get cancer and sometimes nobody ever knows
why. Finally she had gone to see a *hataalii*. He had performed a ceremony for her, not one so elaborate as a Night
Chant, but one that had greatly calmed her and made her
feel her body's harmony was restored.

In the interest of saving time I scheduled her for a
lumpectomy and axillary dissection. A couple of days later,
during a procedure on another patient, I got a beep on my
pager. It was Carolyn telling me she had decided: "I want to
go through with it."

On a cold morning in January, I stood at the sink for a long time before washing my hands with the prep soap. I began my own small ceremony, clearing my mind of all thoughts and letting balance and peace take their place. I thought about the medicine of the night and fire and stars, and I touched my silver bear necklace. My pulse slowed as my mind focused. I envisioned myself walking in the bear's body, breathing his warm breath, and I began to feel his strength. It is an image I use often to clear my mind. Soon, I thought as I held the warm metal, I would put my hands into the body of Carolyn Yazzie and remove her cancerous tumor.

▲▲▲▲

After the nurses prepped Carolyn with Betadine, the bright orange solution that cleans the skin, I performed the lumpectomy. I excised the original biopsy site and removed the surrounding breast tissue with electrocautery, a wandlike instrument that works like a knife to electrically incise tissue.

"Guess what?" asked Sue, my colleague who was assisting me, as I exchanged the bovie for a scalpel. Someone had put on a Bonnie Raitt tape and a verse of "Scared to Run Out of Time" was playing for the second time.

"What?" I said.

"Joe and I are getting married," she said. "He asked me last night."

"All right, Sue!" Joe Botticelli was her boyfriend, a dark-haired, mustached engineer with a good sense of humor who had adored Sue from the moment they met. I felt happy that she had broken this good news during Carolyn's surgery. The atmosphere seemed good. A nice feeling filled the OR. Everyone seemed to be smiling under their surgical masks.

I performed the axillary dissection by making another small incision under Carolyn's arm and removing a mass of the lymph nodes that drain the breast tissue. Sue helped me close up the subcutaneous tissue over a small drain, and then close the skin with sutures.

The scar where Carolyn's tumor was extracted would become a thin line, like one a pencil might draw, on the right side of her breast. Later Carolyn's radiation therapist in Albuquerque complimented her on it. I remember thinking at the time that the way a patient heals has as much to do with the patient as it does with surgical skills. Carolyn was young and her body quickly healed itself. Both her lumpectomy and the lymph node biopsies came back negative. Yet I couldn't help thinking that the serene energy in the OR had a hand in making things go especially smoothly.

"I think we caught it," I told Carolyn on a snowy January morning when she came in for a final examination, wearing mittens, a hat, and a bulky coat made of Pendleton wool. I felt such relief. Many stories that surgeons tell have unhappy endings. But so far Carolyn's was not to be one of them. She left my office with an expression of calm and repose I had not seen before. They say that doctors feel very separate from the lives of their patients, but it had not been so for me. I had felt connected to Carolyn's situation and very helpless about improving the way her disease was treated by those in her life.

And as she left, I knew that back in Windowrock, where the wind had sculpted rock in the hills into smooth silky forms, the most famous of which is the one the town is named for, nobody would be afraid to eat Carolyn Yazzie's fry bread anymore.

▲▲▲▲

Not long after Carolyn's surgery, a wonderful thing happened at the Gallup Indian Medical Center. For a few months our intensive care unit was being modernized and rebuilt; during that period we had to work out of a makeshift ICU that was set up next to a suite of operating rooms.

One day the ICU nurses called all the doctors at the hospital to the new ICU. When I got there, I saw why. One of the nurses' relatives was a medicine man, and the nurses had invited him to perform a blessing ceremony over the new ICU—a Navajo blessing, over a place where Navajos came when they were very, very sick. Many had died in the room, so the blessing was very important and would abolish any lingering *ch'įįndis*.

The *hataałii* stood next to his wife. They were both dressed in traditional clothing. Inside, patients lay in their beds in various states of consciousness, some of them glancing over, a tiny bit curious about what was about to happen. Some had suffered strokes. Others had cancer. Still others had illnesses associated with alcoholism like acute pancreatitis and kidney disease. In his hand the *hataałii* held a feather and a bowl of sacred water. He began to sing.

Amid the brand-new computers with their readouts of heart tracings, the oxygen equipment that fed patients vital gases, and the IV bags that dripped nourishment and medicine into patients' veins, among the new, special ICU beds and the most high-tech equipment in the whole hospital, the ancient man walked. He stepped over to the row of doctors and waved an eagle feather. Over each of our bodies, he twirled the feather and then sprinkled us with water. His voice rang out, rhythmic and atonal, that familiar sound of Navajo chant, a series of glottal stops and resonating notes that seemed to come from deep inside. I remembered this healing sound from the furthest reaches of my childhood. This ceremony medicine could make it possible for Navajo patients to feel safe being treated in the new ICU. I shut my eyes and let the rattle and hum of his voice enter my bones.

Although my family had visited medicine men and consulted them for various problems, as an adult I'd felt hesitant to go myself. I am not sure exactly why. Maybe it was because I am half-Anglo, or perhaps I felt a bit embarrassed and ashamed that I did not speak Navajo well. A part of me was afraid that he would tell me I am not "Navajo enough" to receive or learn about a traditional cure. Yet if I wanted to improve my own surgical practice, I needed to know more about traditional medicine.

Standing there in the ICU, I decided that I *would* go to visit a medicine man. But I wanted a reason; my visit to a *hataałii* would have to occur in its own time.

▲▲▲▲

Chapter Seven

SPIRITUAL SURGERY

About halfway between Gallup and Crownpoint is a place known locally as Satan's Pass, a sinister-looking section of turns and twists in the road where sharp cliffs loom ominously above. Yet that winter morning it looked serenely innocent under a smooth cover of new snow. Listening to the radio fade in and out, I drove through a starkly clean, white world on my way to meet the patients at the Crownpoint clinic, where I made periodic visits.

When I walked into the clinic room, she was already there, waiting. Somehow seeing Dezbah Tsosie calmed me. Dressed in cotton slacks and top, with a print kerchief tied beneath her chin in an old-fashioned style that Navajo grandmothers often wear, she sat quietly on the examining table with her hands folded neatly in her lap. Although she was only in her late forties, her face was etched with an elaborate wizardry of deep lines. "*Yáat'ééh*, Mrs. Tsosie," I said.

"*Yáat'ééh*, Doctor," she said.

"What's bothering you today?" I asked, after glancing over her chart.

She told me right away that she had been having sharp abdominal pains after eating. Immediately a familiar bell rang in my head. I had encountered gallbladder problems so often by then, I could probably diagnose them in my sleep.

"Where?" I asked her. "Can you show me?"

She pointed to her body, a place on the right side, just underneath her rib cage.

"Is it worse after eating meat and fried foods?"

She nodded. After she lay down, I unbuttoned her shirt, careful to expose only a small part of her body, and manually examined her abdomen. She had a mild tenderness just beneath her right rib cage.

Mrs. Tsosie told me she lived in Ganado and that her clan was the *Kin Yaa'aanii,* or the towering house clan, and that she was born for the *Tsi'naajinii* clan. "Then we are related," I told her. "My father's people are *Tsi'naajinii.*"

I explained to her that, based on the results of a few tests, we would have to do surgery to remove her gallbladder.

"Yes, I know." She nodded.

"How do you know that, Dezbah?" She looked down, as though she were speaking directly to the diseased organ within her.

"The *hataałii* told me," she said. "He says I have gallstones. He told me to come here and get them removed."

I smiled to myself—medicine men can be very astute at diagnosis.

"If we do remove it," I said, "you will have a few little scars on your belly—here, here, and here." I pointed at my own abdomen, to illustrate where the tiny incisions for the laparoscopic instruments would be made.

Again she nodded knowingly. Maybe he had told her that, too.

▲▲▲▲

Navajos frequently get large gallstones and diseased gall-bladders. The reason is that the ancient diet of grains, beans, and limited meat has been replaced in the matter of a generation by a diet of lipids, cholesterol, and sugars. Furthermore, the extremely active former lifestyle of herding sheep and goats and farming is disappearing. This rapid change in diet and lifestyle has had a bad effect on health. As in the *bilagáana* world, television has become the hearth in many modern Navajo homes. But Navajos make bad couch potatoes. I could see this in the diseased gallbladders of patients like Dezbah Tsosie.

Navajo medicine men seem to know these things, too. Patients like Dezbah often say the medicine man told them they have diabetes, gallstones, or other diseases, and we do the ultrasounds and other diagnostic tests and sure enough, they are right. I often get such "referrals." Many believe that "white men's medicine" is better at curing "white men's diseases"—sick gallbladders and diabetes being the most obvious examples. Sometimes the *hataałii* will say: "The white people's doctors can help you with this—they know how to fix this."

They are right—we do. Like many surgeons, we use a nickname for the most common operation we perform at GIMC, as though it were an old friend of ours: the "lap-chole" (pronounced "lap kolee"), short for laparoscopic cholecystectomy. In layman's terms the lap-choly is the removal of the gallbladder using sophisticated, tiny, state-of-the-art instruments.

We always worked in teams of two during the surgery, which meant that I worked with Tim, Sue, or another staff surgeon, sometimes performing as many as three lap-cholies a day and assisting on a fourth. A few years earlier, when

I started medical school, the technology for the procedure hadn't even existed. By the time I arrived in Gallup, we were removing more than three hundred gallbladders laparoscopically a year—a very high volume for a hospital of our size.

I often described the gallbladder to patients like Dezbah as an auxiliary organ. It sits to the side of the liver, which provides the intestines with bile, a digestive enzyme that aids in breaking down food. The food has already been partially digested by acids in the stomach. The gallbladder gives it one more little shot. In some people the gallbladder develops "stones" that block the ducts through which the bile is delivered. When these ducts become blocked, bile builds up inside, and very serious infections can develop. When they do, patients can experience a great deal of pain. I encourage patients at this stage to have their gallbladders removed.

Although this small pickle-shaped organ helps in digestion, a person can live a normal life without one, just as they can without an appendix or a spleen. Now that we can remove gallbladders laparoscopically, the procedure is even less traumatic; all we leave behind are four tiny wounds.

During surgery in the darkened sanctum of the OR, I would watch the video monitor as the laparoscopic equipment moved through shiny pink, blue, and orange tissue laced with purple capillaries and white braids of fatty tissue. Lit up on the large surgical video monitor, the inside of the body can be exquisite. Sometimes the familiar shapes of the liver's lobes, the gallbladder, the stomach, the spleen, and the pancreas, and the delicate, curving arches of the duodenum, colon, and small intestines look strange and surreal, like Expressionist art. If a capillary is cut when the laparoscopic equipment punctures tissues to delve further inside the body, the screen blooms with red lilies of blood. When the gallbladder is punctured, an inky fluid pours out. Using tiny suctioning tools and fancy cautery wands, the blood and bile are magically removed, and the shiny tissue beneath reappears.

Sometimes as we were working, I'd look around at my colleagues, costumed in surgical masks and scrubs. We used these new tools so easily (they hadn't even existed six years earlier), and they gave us untold new powers of perception. In essence, they allowed us to operate and see with tiny cameras in a sacred, secret place—the unopened human body. This never ceased to amaze me. We have instruments and cameras so small that they fit into a half-inch slit underneath an umbilicus. With laparoscopic technology, a scope can be sent in to view a troubled area, a procedure can be accomplished, or a diseased organ excised, with less damage to muscles and skin, less pain, and a quicker recovery period than in older forms of surgery.

Although a surgical procedure focuses on a single organ, I always tried to stay aware of the whole person—organs, mind, and spirit, the harmony of their entire being.

> *I am opening a person.*
> *I am putting my hands inside their body.*
> *I am touching places so private that this person has*
>   *never even seen them themselves.*

At Gallup I was gaining access to the most personal territory in the world, and I was becoming more and more careful not to disrespect this territory. It was an honor to have the trust of my Navajo patients.

Whether I was looking at the shiny fascia covering the person's muscles, or the whitish peritoneum that lines some organs and the abdominal cavity like a fine tissue, or a swollen, infected gallbladder or appendix, what I often felt was awe and reverence. As surgeons, we travel to these places on a special visa that makes us invited guests in a secret, forbidden country.

To our patients, the surgery we did was magical and, I had come to realize, made us the modern-day equivalent of shamans. It was as though, by virtue of our skills, we had special powers, and people sometimes looked to us to transcend the possible and even extend human life. For Navajos, healer and holy man were merged, and doctor and priest were one and the same. A *haataɫii* did not treat a person's liver or spleen or appendix—although, as in the case of Dezbah Tsosie, they could be perfectly aware that a problem resided in such an organ. But they did not isolate a part from the whole. Their medicine was for the whole human creature—body, mind, and spirit, their community, and even the larger world. I had come to think of this philosophy as a gift that could be given by Navajos to the medical world.

Indians had already brought much to the medical world. Their contributions to pharmacology alone were staggering, as Western medicine had adopted many Indian cures. Quinine, used to treat malaria, had been brought to Western attention by the indigenous people of Peru; a bark from an evergreen tree was given by the Hurons to the French explorer Jacques Cartier to treat scurvy; Indians taught Europeans how to use the bark of the willow to cure pain—which eventually led to the development of aspirin. Early Indian healers lanced boils, set bones, gave enemas, and invented bulb syringes—they even had "surgeons" who could amputate. I wanted to find a way to make the medical world equally conscious of the philosophical contributions to healing of Native people, which were just as valuable.

But balance, harmony, and wholeness were not the emphasis of my own field, as I was constantly reminded when I went to professional meetings or read surgical and medical journals. Transplant surgeons on current frontiers of surgical technology illustrated this as they "harvested" organs from the dead and placed them, like spare parts, into the sick. But the best surgeons didn't operate on gallbladders or spleens or hearts, they operated on the people who owned them. People with children, jobs, interests, and beliefs. They operated on lives. On people like Dezbah Tsosie.

At its best, performing surgery could itself be a spiritual experience. When done correctly, all the actions are fluid, and no movement is wasted. The surgical team works in concert, and the result is like choreography. Yet we repair bodies and save lives.

When a Navajo patient told me they needed a ceremony before surgery, I would adjust the schedule of their surgery to allow time for it. I had noticed that the *hataałii*, sings, and ceremonies like the Yeibechei calmed patients considerably, and a calm patient was a much better candidate for surgery. Their heart and blood pressure rates were lower. They were relaxed. The *hataałii* did subtle things that we had not quantitatively measured. It is said that they could help patients control their own bleeding. I had no reason not to believe it. New technologies, like biofeedback, were helping us understand that the mind can indeed control the body. New research has even shown that the mind is able to positively or negatively influence the immune system, and our body's ability to fight against cancers and infections. Medicine men were capable of working through channels that we in Western medicine did not yet understand. Navajo healers clearly practiced a viable and real medicine that worked with the patient's mind as well as their body.

One Native American writer and healer, Brooke Medicine Eagle, points out that the word *heal* comes from the same root as *whole* and *holiness*. For Navajos, wholeness and holiness are the same thing. The system of life is one interconnected whole. Everything is related, according to Navajo beliefs—it is an organic and integrated way of looking at the world. The causes and cures for illness are woven into everything else.

Although we try to make surgery go smoothly and to reach the desired outcome in a timely fashion, not everything that happens in the OR is predictable. Right before the eyes of the doctors, nurses, and technicians, lives come into being and fade into cardiac flat lines. Surgery is enormously stressful, filled with moments of victory and defeat. Every movement requires precision and acute attention.

The Navajo word *na'agizh* means "surgery," but it translates literally as "to cut open." Many traditional Navajo people are opposed to the idea since it goes against the Navajo philosophy of the sacred, natural order and beauty of the universe. Many Navajos cannot understand how it could be beneficial to cut open a human body and remove a part of it, disturbing the harmony of the whole. When I first decided to become a surgeon, I had to face the fact that some Navajos would question my methods of healing, and might wonder why I chose a surgical field. Part of the answer was that many Navajos had already had surgery, and many more would certainly need it, and I wanted them to have the option of a Navajo surgeon.

Just before Dezbah Tsosie's surgery, her cousin Bertha Sam said she wanted to talk to me. "Dezbah wants her organs, you know, after you take them out." I nodded. I had expected it. Such requests from Navajo patients who have had their appendix, gallbladder, or other body tissue surgically removed by now seemed normal to me. They even wanted infected tissue back. It was commonplace for patients to leave the hospital with a line of new black stitches sewn on their abdomen and a small paper bag in their hand, the contents of which had resided inside them several days earlier. It was the same for any body part: hair, skin, nails, even the skin for a circumcision— all are carefully protected. It is believed that Navajo witches could obtain these objects and use them in ceremonies to cause harm to the person they belong to.

▲▲▲▲

A few weeks after the snowy morning when I first met Dezbah Tsosie in Crownpoint, I found myself facing her again. The snow that clothed the pass had melted, replaced

by a searing high wind that pushed the car to the left side of
the road with fury. Once again, as I drove out to see how she
and a few of my other patients were doing, Satan's Pass had
taken on its demonic personality, baring its fangs.

On a cold winter morning a few days earlier, I'd performed
Dezbah Tsosie's lap-choly with Tim's assistance, and there
were no high-drama moments or surprises. Everything went
smoothly, and at the end I presented her husband, Ernie
Tsosie, with a paper bag with the requested contents. On
that windy morning she returned to the Crownpoint clinic for
her postop checkup.

"How are you, Dezbah?" I asked.

"Pretty good," she said. I lifted her shirt and examined the
small wounds on her abdomen. They had become an assort-
ment of tiny creases with small scales, like dash marks. She'd
had a ceremony, she said, and the *hataalii* believed she was
healed.

"I believe that you are healed now, too, Dezbah," I said.
She had very little tenderness in her abdomen, and her overall complexion was healthier. "You can tell the medicine man
I agree with him completely. In fact, I don't think you'll even
need to come back, unless this begins to bother you or gets
infected or sore."

As I walked her to the door, she smiled at me. "Doctor?"
she asked. I turned to her. *"Ahéhee'."*

It was the Navajo word for "thank you."

Chapter Eight

▲▲▲▲

THE "NAVAJO PLAGUE"

*Many Navajos have strayed from traditional
beliefs and practices in healthy living and
respect for nature. As a result, illness has
taken the lives of innocent people.*

—NAVAJO MEDICINE MAN,
*quoted on a poster sponsored
by the Indian Health Service
and the Navajo Division
of Health*

It seemed more like an episode from *The X-Files*
than real life. "You know that woman you operated
on, the one you sent home a week ago?" a doctor at
the hospital asked Sue and me one spring morning
in 1993. We both nodded.

"She died this morning in Crownpoint, at the
clinic," he said.

We looked at one another in shock.

How could Florena Woody have died? The
twenty-four-year-old woman from the tiny community of Littlewater had complained of a stuffy nose,
a dry cough, aches, and little else. From all the
available evidence, it looked like an ordinary case
of the flu to Sue, who had examined her at the
Crownpoint clinic.

In fact, Florena had come in not because of her cold symptoms but for a follow-up examination for the surgery that Sue had performed, with my assistance, a week earlier. We had taken her to the OR for biliary colic and gallstones. She underwent a lap-choly and her surgery was uneventful. As far as we could tell, everything had gone perfectly smoothly.

During her follow-up exam, Sue had seen no evidence of fever, the incision was healing nicely, and Florena was eating well. By all our surgical and medical standards, Sue had every reason to believe that, despite some cold symptoms, Florena was fine.

After the examination, Sue gave her the standard advice— get some rest, drink plenty of fluids, and come back if she got a fever or didn't feel better the next day.

What could we have missed or done wrong? Why on earth had this healthy, athletic young woman died?

In the 1990s, the fear of malpractice suits is strong among all physicians, and our colleague's voice had held an uneasy note. The subtext to his comment was a hidden sentence that I imagined went something like: *Okay, what really happened during her surgery?*

At the time of Florena Woody's death, I was comfortable and happy in my practice at GIMC. Gallup had become my home. Sue and I had operated hundreds of times together. In the OR our communication had become natural, fluid, and fun.

I respected Sue. She and Tim weren't like other doctors at remote facilities who were simply fulfilling contracts that would pay back a medical loan, or who could not find work elsewhere. They had both chosen to work with Native people and previously had worked at other Indian hospitals.

Sue and I had done procedures together so many times that it seemed as if we could read each other's mind. It was a surgical version of the phenomenon that happens when you have known someone for such a long time that you begin to say the same thing at the same time.

That is why we were so surprised when we heard about Florena Woody. All day we waited to hear more about her case. What would her autopsy reveal? Maybe—worst-case scenario—her sudden illness had been due to a severe case of septic shock as a result of our surgery. An ominous feeling hung in the air.

All day we kept running into each other in the hallways and nervously asking: "Heard anything?"

"No, I thought you would have heard something."

Then the story came in.

Florena Woody had shown up in Crownpoint in severe respiratory distress and hypoxic—with too little oxygen in her blood. She'd died a few hours later.

To a person untrained in medicine, it is difficult to describe the impact this news had on us. Such symptoms were extremely rare.

Furthermore, I had never before lost a young, healthy patient after a purely elective procedure. I thought of Florena's family and all the things she might have done with the rest of her life. Each time I thought about her—young and smart, carelessly swinging her feet off the edge of the examining table with a certain girlishness, smiling brightly—I felt an unnameable sensation, part pain and part fear mixed with internal searching. I went over and over her surgical procedure in my mind, searching for clues as to what might have gone wrong. But each time I came up with nothing.

When a patient signs a surgical release form, they entrust the surgeon with their most precious possession, their body. It is a contract of the highest order. No legal agreement, no other human contract, carries the same weight.

According to the Hippocratic oath, the physician's responsibility is to do no harm, but that is just the beginning. Surgeons are also required to find and repair malfunctioning, remove disease, ease discomfort, improve overall health, and extend life. Unlike other physicians, surgeons cannot carry out their jobs without some element of risk.

The risks in laparoscopic surgery are compounded by the fact that in this kind of surgery, we cannot feel things with our own hands. We operate through tiny keyhole incisions and place instruments through them that do the touching and dissecting for us. The sensory feedback is not as perfect as if we were making the cuts with our hands. In fact, some older surgeons were initially reluctant to incorporate laparoscopic surgery into their practices for this very reason: they trusted the ten fingers they had always relied on.

Our main concern about the laparoscopic cholecystectomy we performed on Florena Woody was the possibility of a bile duct leak. The common bile duct is a tube that drains bile from the liver. The gallbladder drains into the common bile duct through another small tube called a cystic duct, which must be tied off or clipped and divided when removing the gallbladder. We thought that, when we removed her gallbladder, a cystic duct leak or a common bile duct injury might have occurred. Such a leak could have let bile spill into the abdomen, which could in turn have caused a rapidly spreading infection throughout the body known as sepsis or septic shock. This conclusion is rare and difficult to anticipate, and there had been no symptoms of it in Florena Woody. I felt it simply hadn't happened. But what else could have caused her to die?

By the next day people at GIMC were even more alarmed. Sue and I were asked a number of times about Florena Woody's condition during and right after her surgery. Then the surgical staff met and discussed her case. The autopsy results came in.

Apparently she had died of "catastrophic asphyxiation," meaning her lungs had filled with fluid until she could no longer breathe. Florena Woody had drowned in her own body fluids.

When we got the next piece of news, everything stopped: Merrill Bahe, Florena Woody's nineteen-year-old fiancé, had become similarly ill on the day of Florena's funeral. He had been brought to the GIMC emergency room in full respiratory and cardiac arrest and died shortly thereafter.

Whatever Florena Woody had, her boyfriend had had it, too. And it was something the likes of which nobody had ever seen.

I have to admit to an initial sense of relief for Sue and me—we were not after all associated with the cause of Ms. Woody's death. But our concern also intensified, since the cause of two rapid deaths was now even harder to comprehend. Could it be some strange new ailment? we wondered. Had Sue and I and our surgical staff been exposed to it during the surgery? New and unexplained illnesses, like the Ebola virus and Marburg virus in Africa, pop up from time to time all over the world, baffling physicians and terrifying the general public. Could this be one of them?

During the next week more cases of what was by then being called the "mystery flu" appeared in Crownpoint and in Zuni, and then, quite inexplicably, more deaths occurred in young, healthy people.

These were people in their twenties and thirties, complaining of aches and fevers, trouble breathing, and sore throats and bellies. They should have been treatable with fluids and aspirin, not being prepared for funerals. In reaction the hospitals were flooded with frightened patients and people who had heard of or were related to the deceased, most of whom had nothing more than the usual colds and flus. Everyone in the hospital was quite baffled, and there was talk of little else.

At this point, I would later learn, a Navajo physician consulted a medicine man about the ailment. Dr. Ben Muneta, a Navajo who happened to work for the CDC, visited Andy Natonabah, a *hataałii*. Natonabah told him the illness was caused by an excess of rainfall, which had caused the piñon trees to bear too much fruit.

The unexpectedly large harvest of piñon nuts was a significant deviation from the natural harmony of the world.

According to the *hataałii*, this was what was causing people to become sick.

While the epidemiologists were looking for the solution in their microscopes, the *hataałii* had looked to the macro level—disturbed natural patterns in the universe. I pondered the *hataałii*'s words. How could excessive piñon nuts cause a life-threatening illness? Why hadn't someone on staff isolated and identified the illness yet?

Within a few more days, officials from the Centers for Disease Control descended upon our little corner of the world. National newspapers had arrived with them and were calling the ailment the Navajo plague. All around the reservation, doctors were put on alert.

Both Tom Brokaw and Peter Jennings described the "Navajo mystery virus" on the national nightly news.

A reporter from *The New York Times* wrote: "Perhaps never before has a mystery held the Navajo Nation and surrounding towns in such a tight vise as has the devastating flulike illness that has swept through the Four Corners region of New Mexico and Arizona. . . . Every possible theory, from the sacred to the mundane, has been offered to explain the ailment, called acute respiratory distress syndrome."

The *Times* reported that at least a dozen laboratories were taking part in the inquiry, among them teams at the Indian Health Service, the Navajo Nation, the New Mexico Department of Health, the Centers for Disease Control, the Los Alamos National Laboratory, and Sandia National Laboratory.

I remembered the case of the man with the porcupine quill in his intestine when I had first arrived in Gallup. This flu, too, seemed to defy all our medical understanding.

Then more stories came in from all around the reservation and as far away as Farmington, New Mexico, and Phoenix, Arizona: People were refusing to serve Navajos in restaurants. Individuals all over were canceling their vacations to the Southwest. The virus was being framed as a Navajo disease. The national media jumped to the conclusion that it was *because they were Navajo* that these individuals had contracted it. The ugly stereotypes of "dirty Indian," "bad Indian," "unhygienic Indian" were rearing their heads again. The logic went something like this: *It must be the way those Navajos live that is causing them to sicken and die.*

I was often aware of that stereotype. Even in my most personal life, it had affected me. I'd often found myself fighting the urge to clean things and clean them twice.

When racial prejudice rose up in the midst of the health crisis I felt a familiar wave of despair. From time to time such bigotry disappears, and the world feels as if it is progressing toward mutual cultural respect—but it always seems to come back. Any dominant culture seems to accuse its subordinate culture of lack of cleanliness. The Germans decried the supposed unclean practices of Jews in the 1930s. White people accused blacks of uncouth and unclean living. And Indians historically often have been described as dirty.

Alarmed by this negative publicity, Navajos struck back. The disease was brought to the reservation by white tourists, they said. By this time, they protested, seven whites and one Hispanic had contracted it as well, so it could no longer be called a Navajo virus.

But the illness continued, regardless of the culture war it had propagated. During the next few weeks eleven more people on the reservation died and seven others began experiencing the flulike symptoms of the mystery illness. The explanatory theories were spreading with a speed almost as rapid, among them that the deaths were caused when the government sprayed peyote plants in order to deter Navajos from eating their hallucinogenic buttons; an unidentified bacterium was secreting "lethal proteins" in people's lungs; it was a version of Epstein-Barr syndrome, AIDS, streptococcus, or staphylococcus pneumonia, anthrax, or bubonic plague.

My favorite explanation was the one about Fort Wingate, a storage facility for missiles near Gallup. Some people were saying that radioactive materials had leaked from the weapons there and sunk into the groundwater, and that was what was making people sick. The illness was a conspiracy theorist's field day.

Late one afternoon in May, as I was getting ready to leave GIMC for the day, I was called to see a patient who complained of severe abdominal pain in the lower right quadrant.

Betty Cowboy, a Navajo silversmith in her late forties with eight children, showed up with a white blood cell count of twenty-eight thousand. Such a high white count is something we rarely see unless the patient has a severe infection, such as a ruptured appendix. As I examined her, pressing on her abdomen in search of signs of infection or distress, I asked her how she was feeling.

In broken English combined with Navajo, she described herself as "feeling achy all over, with an ache in my head" as well as experiencing abdominal pain. But as I pressed her abdomen, it didn't feel tender, as though anything were wrong there.

When I said I didn't think Betty Cowboy had appendicitis, the internal medicine physicians challenged me. I took a deep breath. I knew I had better be right, and I decided to admit her overnight into the intensive care unit for close observation. When I called in later that evening to check up on my patients, the ICU nurse said, "Ms. Cowboy seems fine. No sign of escalating fevers or discomfort. We think she can go home in the morning." I went to sleep that night planning what I would say the next day to the doctors who had challenged my diagnosis.

But at 6:00 A.M. my beeper went off. It was the ICU nurse on duty.

Betty Cowboy was having trouble breathing, her oxygen saturation had dropped, and her fever had spiked to 104. I got out of bed, threw on some clothes, and grabbed a cup of coffee.

By the time I got to the hospital, she was on oxygen and

hooked to a ventilator. Her condition was upgraded to serious. By 9:00 A.M., her breathing had become labored, infiltrates were visible on her chest X-ray, and her lungs were turning white and filling with fluid. At that point everyone agreed that it looked like the mystery virus. The air ambulance team was called, and they strapped her to a gurney and rushed her to an emergency helicopter. She was flown to the University of New Mexico Hospital in Albuquerque, where researchers were trying to piece together clues about the virus with their better diagnostic tools.

The call came from an ICU nurse later that night, just as I was cooking a pot of posole for Grandma's and my dinner: Betty Cowboy had died.

My throat tightened. The day before she'd spoken about the children she was raising. She'd told me about her little boy who had seemed to skip the crawling stage and simply stood up and began to walk one day. It seemed impossible that his mother was no longer in this world. What sort of disease snatches someone so fast? And had I possibly come into contact with the germs? I'd treated Betty in an airless examining room and had palpated her abdomen without gloves. A shiver of fear zipped up my spine.

By this time one theory had emerged as the dominant one held by the CDC. Although it had never been associated with death by asphyxiation, the mystery disease was believed to be a hantavirus, contracted from the droppings or urine of infected deer mice. Such droppings had been found in the trailer where Florena Woody and Merrill Bahe had lived. The hantavirus strain was found in their tissues and analyzed after their autopsies, as well as in the tissues of other mystery virus patients. Furthermore, the deer mouse population had surged that fall, biologists said, in response to a huge windfall crop of piñon nuts.

The realization spread through me like a chill: The rainfall *had* caused the piñon crop to be larger than usual. The piñon crop in turn, had fed the mice, whose droppings had spread the disease. The world had indeed fallen out of balance.

Weeks earlier the medicine man Natonabah had given the very same explanation. He had shown Muneta an old photograph of a sand painting with a mouse painted into it. Muneta had stared at it long and hard. Natonabah told him that many years ago such a sickness had occurred and that the sand painting had been used to treat it.

"Look to the mouse," Ben Muneta was told. He had taken this information back to the CDC. This piece of information was what led the CDC to consider the mouse as the source of the virus.

On June 7, the Associated Press ran an article that confirmed it:

"Health officials said today that the latest findings suggested that they were on the right track in their theory that a mysterious, deadly disease may be caused by a virus found in rodent droppings. . . . No new cases of the illness were reported over the weekend. Of eighteen confirmed cases, seven in New Mexico and four in Arizona have been fatal. Most victims have been Navajos."

Unfortunately Navajos seem to be susceptible to many diseases that have been all but eradicated in most parts of the country. They have frequent tuberculosis and sporadic cases of plague. Epidemics like measles and meningitis, easily controlled elsewhere, can spread like wildfire on the reservation.

The reasons are partly economic. Because of the extreme poverty in some places on the reservation, poor nutrition is ever present, leading to increased susceptibility to disease. Also, many Navajos live in remote areas where the well water isn't always sanitary. The reasons are also partly cultural. Navajos frequently hunt deer and elk, which are associated with diseases carried by ticks, like Rocky Mountain fever. Navajos often work closely with animals, like sheep and cattle, since animal husbandry is a main occupation. This kind

of residence and work pattern is associated with certain
other diseases as well.

"Scarlet fever was good for me," said my grandmother
Grace Cupp ironically as she recalled an epidemic that
struck the reservation when she was a child. "It saved my
life." She had been taken to a hospital where she was quar-
antined for several weeks. When she returned home she
found that her mother and many of her relatives had died in
the great influenza epidemic of 1919, which swept through
the Navajo reservation, taking thousands of lives.

I cannot imagine what it must have been like for a little
girl to undergo such an experience, separated from her
family, being all alone, and coming home to find her entire
world devastated and her mother dead. Her father had re-
married shortly thereafter, to her mother's sister, and she
grew up having her aunt as her second mother and her cousins as new brothers and sisters.

In my own life, I have seen epidemics of plague and
measles on the reservation. I think back upon the hantavirus
often, especially when I go to the Crownpoint clinic and see
the Indian Health Service poster that hangs in every examining room. Four Ways to Protect Your Family From the Hantavirus, it reads.

The poster tells the story that medicine people and Navajo
elders tell about the years 1918 and 1933 when above-
average rainfall and year-round availability of piñon nuts led
to an increase in the rodent population. There were many
deaths at the time, perhaps caused by a hantavirus. Oral tradition and the practice of tribal storytelling have kept this
history alive. Maybe my grandmother's mother was a victim
of a hantavirus, too.

The poster continues: "Traditional Navajo belief, which
Western medicine now supports, says that rodents and humans should live separately because of this concern for illness. Today it is known that this illness is the hantavirus
infection, which results when viral particles from infected

rodents are inhaled." It offers guidelines for cleaning and disinfecting homes and workplaces where rodents have lived.

I thought back to the principles of the Beauty Way and the teaching that illness is a result of life out of balance. The hantavirus was a classic example of that principle, only this time it wasn't human life that was out of balance; "rain life," "piñon tree life," and "mouse life" had fallen out of balance and caused humans to become ill.

Many generations ago, astonishingly, the keen observational skills of Navajo people and their harmony with the natural world had led them to observe relationships in the environment and animal world that had, in the end, helped the CDC narrow their search to the mouse. Our ancestors were astute epidemiologists!

In the weeks that followed, I read the papers daily for some article acknowledging the role that traditional beliefs had played in finding the key to the mystery, but I found none, only more confirmation of the orgins of the disease. "There is no person-to-person spread of hantavirus," Dr. Bruce Tempest, a director at GIMC, was quoted explaining. "You have to catch it from the mice themselves or from their dropings or urine."

It wasn't the deer mice who were ultimately responsible. Ask the medicine men. They'd known all along how life had fallen out of balance. It was the rain.

Chapter Nine

▲▲▲▲

TWO WEDDINGS

Then came the Earth Woman,
Nahosdzan'esdza. First Man told her that she
was to be the wife of the Sky. She would face
the East and her husband over her would face
the West. And whenever Fog covered the
Earth they would know the Sky had visited
Nahosdzan'esdza.

—NAVAJO STORY

I learned to expect the unexpected.

After the hantavirus scare and the other rare medical conditions I'd seen, as well as the stories my patients told of being witched and stalked by skinwalkers, I realized I would have to adjust to the unpredictability of practicing medicine in our corner of the world. Strange and rare medical events seemed more or less par for the course in Gallup. Odd things occurred almost daily. I decided simply to relax and be open.

One such thing that happened in 1993 changed my personal life forever. It was not a skinwalker visitation, nor a porcupine quill in an abdomen, nor a woman struck by cancer-causing lightning, but it was just as strange and mysterious. It was strange because it was unexpected, taking me entirely by surprise.

During a routine appendectomy one afternoon, I looked up to ask for a clamp. A pair of unfamiliar, startlingly blue eyes gazed at me over the blue surgical mask. They belonged to a young man in an Army Special Forces medic training group. The army assigned a few of these teams to our hospital to learn clinical skills, so every month or so a new crew showed up, scrubbed in, and learned a little from us about surgery and anesthesia. The Special Forces guys filed into and out of our lives with little real effect. We were all very cordial, exchanging pleasantries and a lot of smiles, but we never really got to know one another.

That afternoon the owner of the bright eyes and I struck up a light conversation during the surgery. *Okay, newcomer interview,* I thought.

"So where did you say you're from, Jon?" I asked, suctioning some fluid out of the patient's abdomen.

"Salt Lake City," he replied over the bright *shhhh* sound of evacuating liquid.

Borrrring.

"Have you always lived there?" I asked, glancing at the video screen to check the position of the gallbladder.

"No, before that I lived in Kansas."

And I thought Utah was boring.

Later, when he appeared in the hallway in regular clothing, I saw he was also the owner of a head of closely cropped, military-style blond hair, a matching mustache, and an easygoing, comfortable demeanor. I took him in with passing interest, the way I'd skim a magazine, then went on to see my next surgery patient.

Over the next few days, the young Special Forces intern seemed to blend into our surroundings. He was quiet, polite, and often at hand to help out in the OR. It was easy to incorporate his presence, and he didn't plague us with annoying questions.

Several days later, while driving home from the hospital after a grueling morning—too many cases and not enough surgeons had had me in mask, goggles, and scrubs since seven o'clock—my beeper went off.

Not again, I thought, imagining another emergency case calling me back to the OR. On my cellular phone, I dialed the number that my pager listed and stared covetously at the McDonald's drive-through line across the street. It had been a long time since breakfast—a cup of coffee and a slice of toast.

"Hi," a voice answered. Not your average response to a beeper.

"Hi?" I asked.

"Yeah, hi," it repeated. "It's Jon. I was wondering if you'd be free for lunch tomorrow."

I exhaled my relief: it wasn't an emergency, a trauma patient, or a coding patient in the ICU. It was Jon Alvord, the Special Forces student with awesome blue eyes. *Well, well,* I thought.

He can't actually be interested in me, he is so much younger than I am. He must want something else. The thoughts rifled through my mind as I wondered what to say. I was sure the invitation was innocent. Something about those eyes seemed incapable of bullshit.

"Okay," I answered. "Do you want me to invite anyone else along?"

"No, not really," he said. "See you tomorrow."

The next day, after another grueling morning in the OR with a stubborn gallbladder, I met Jon at Earl's, a local favorite diner on the old Route 66, featuring hot chili and roomy booths. It is known for the roaming Navajo artisans who peddle their wares to the diners.

Over big platters of huevos rancheros and large iced teas, Jon Alvord and I spoke casually about this and that, and I found myself responding to him teasingly. First he told me about his hobbies: skydiving, mountain biking, and skiing. He'd also recently tried bungee jumping. "You must like air," I said, "falling through air." *Adventure junkie.*

"I do," he answered. Then I found out two other interesting pieces of information. First, it had taken him two weeks to get up the courage to ask me out. Second, he was twenty-three. I was thirty-four. I thought about the age difference and decided I wouldn't let it bother me. I had known men in their early twenties who were very mature, and I had known men in their thirties and forties who were anything but mature. With a little irritation, I realized that if he were my age and I was his age, society wouldn't even question our relationship.

In my dating career, which had been long and filled with various disappointments, I'd dated all sorts of people: other surgeons, engineers, teachers, and politicians. Most of them, by my own choice, were Native American. Once at Stanford I'd had to cut off a budding relationship with a Navajo man, because we had learned that we belonged to the same clan, which is an absolutely unbreachable taboo.

I had dated men from other tribes as well—Hopi, Jemez, Taos, Santa Domingo—and even a few from more distant regions: Chippewa, Mohawk, Winnebago, Eskimo, and Sioux. Once in a while a long-term relationship would develop but none had ever become permanent.

Although I had occasionally connected with a *bilagáana* man, for most of my life I had considered only Native Americans for serious relationships. It was not prejudice against other races that led me to this preference but pride in my own, and a desire to have a Native partner. I'd seen plenty of mixed marriages work fine, like Valden and his wife, Sue. But I consciously did not want this for myself. For one thing, I knew it would make my children only one-quarter Navajo.

But Jon was quite adorable, and I could see nothing wrong with dating him for a little while. He'd be gone shortly, and in the meantime we clearly enjoyed each other's company. I liked his sense of adventure and his laugh. Surprisingly, he felt right. I was truly amazed that a white man, and one much younger than I, could be such a good fit.

In the next weeks I melted into a bright, happy world with him. We shared pizzas, rented movies, and hiked to the top of the rocky ledge behind my house. He brought many bouquets of flowers. In a particularly postcard moment on a rock-climbing outing, he kissed me before a backdrop of pink and gray clouds.

On the evening before he was scheduled to leave Gallup for another assignment, I got a telephone call from the Gallup Animal Control Center.

"Do you have a dog named Shush?" a man's voice asked.

"Yes."

"Well, she's been hit by a car. We've just picked her up, and she's at the vet now."

She must have gotten out of the yard, I thought. *She's so small, she's probably been hurt bad.*

"I'll be right there," I said, hurriedly. "Thanks." Without even thinking about it, I called Jon and asked him to meet me at the veterinary clinic.

The long-haired yellow terrier had been my friend for almost four years. Her companion, Bouncer, had been a present from my mother's second husband, George Colgan. Life without either of them seemed an empty proposition. Every day they followed Grandmother on her walks on the mesas. They were my family, too.

At the Red Rocks veterinary clinic, the vet said frankly, "Her right leg is smashed. She's gonna lose it."

"What else?" I asked, bracing for even worse news.

"Well, she's lost a lot of blood. We're watching out now for internal injuries. I can't tell you, Lori, if this dog is going to make it, but if she lives and stabilizes, we'll amputate that leg in the morning."

I nodded and looked over at Shush, who was lying on a metal table, hooked up to an IV, a glazed look on her face.

In spite of myself, while standing there in the vet's office with the smell of puppy and frightened cat in the air, I began to cry. "Shusher, little girl, hang in there," I whispered. I wanted to say "I love you," but the veterinary equivalent of an OR nurse ushered me out. A cool smooth hand clasped mine.

Jon and I left the clinic together in his pickup truck. I felt so sad—he was leaving, and now I could lose Shush, too. Emptiness and desperation swirled around me. What did I have in my personal life to really care about? The world I had built for myself was a lonely one. My two sisters had companions. Karen lived with her husband, Billy Sakai, and a darling half-Japanese, one-quarter-Navajo daughter, Cassandra. Robyn had her companion, Verlyn Corbett (who later became her husband), and her son, B.J. My mother had met a new man, too, George, and they had recently married and relocated to Craig, Colorado. She was devoted to him. Only I, alone with Grandma, had no one special, no significant other. Actually Grandma was my significant other, but she was ninety and would not live forever. I couldn't imagine feeling worse. Jon put his arms around me, and I cried some more.

"It'll be okay, Lori," he said.

The comment made me angry. "Okay? How can it be okay? I'm losing you, and now I may lose Shush, too."

"You're not losing me, Lori," he said. I looked up at him. "We're just getting started."

"What?"

"I have a vacation in two weeks, and I'll come back to see you." The words filtered through me. Was this really happening? "I love you, Lori," he said.

My little "noncommittal" relationship with this *bilagáana* boy was suddenly going somewhere fast. His blue eyes looked right into mine, sincerely, startlingly.

Before he left, Jon took several plastic-coated coat hangers. He painted them in bright neon pink and by bending them into the shape of letters, wrote, "Love you forever" with one and "Get well soon" with the other, for Shush. Then he brought me one last present, a crystal vase. I later realized why—it was for all the flowers he would send me while we were apart.

Shush had her surgery the next day, and within a few months she didn't even seem to notice that she had lost her leg—and she was still faster than four-legged Bouncer, who was sweet but rather slow and somewhat obsessed with chasing his own shadow.

Shusher's long hair grew back around the amputation site, and I nicknamed her "my little tripod." Sometimes newcomers would play with her for a few minutes before they'd say: "Hey, this dog only has three legs!"

Jon was now training at Fort Bragg. He'd invited me to visit him there. Under a clear starry sky on Wrightsville Beach in North Carolina, two months to the day from our first date at Earl's diner in Gallup, he asked me to marry him. When I heard the words I was stunned, but I recovered sufficiently to accept his offer, if we could have a yearlong engagement, just to make sure we were making the right decision.

A year after that, in the summer of 1994, I married him—twice. The first wedding was in the hills above Salt Lake City. We exchanged vows under a white canopy in the golden, late-afternoon garden light of a country inn, surrounded by our two families and friends. The second wedding was in a hogan at Churchrock, on the reservation, amidst spears of sunlight speckled with dust. I wore a traditional Navajo velvet shirt, silver belt, skirt, and moccasins, and Jon was dressed like a Navajo groom in a red velvet shirt, with my father's heavy turquoise bracelets and silver belt. Our families were there as well, even some of my more distant relatives and some of my colleagues from the hospital—Sue, Tim, Robyn, and Valden, who brought his wife and baby daughter.

Ernest Becenti, a relative of my family by marriage, was the medicine man who oversaw our traditional Wedding Basket Ceremony in his hogan. The eight-sided traditional structure faces east and the first light of each new day; inside the walls were decorated with Navajo rugs, pottery, and Pendleton blankets. The hushed presence of the circle of people, broken only by an occasional cough or cry of a baby, created a mysterious, sacred atmosphere. Blue cornmeal filled an elaborately woven wedding basket. Ernest Becenti then took out a bag of corn pollen. The basket of cornmeal was placed so that the termination of the weaving faced east. He took a pinch of pollen and sprinkled it in a line from east to west over the cornmeal, then from north to south. Then he made a clockwise corn pollen circle around the basket.

Jon was instructed to take a pinch of the cornmeal at the east end of the line of corn pollen. I did the same, and we placed the cornmeal in our mouths. Then we each took pollen from the south, west, and north and from the center where the two pollen lines crossed, and we ate pollen and blue cornmeal together, symbolizing the joining of our spirits.

Then we passed the basket around in a circle for everyone else in the hogan to eat, until it was gone. We took water from a handmade pottery jar from Acoma Pueblo and poured it over each other's hands.

"You are lucky," Ernest Becenti teased Jon. "If you were Navajo, you would have to bring a lot of sheep and horses for this woman."

After the Basket Ceremony we all drove to the Red Rock Park Center for another reception and dinner. I stepped once more into my white wedding dress, and my sisters put on the beautiful pine-colored gowns they had worn as bridesmaids at my first wedding in Salt Lake City. We danced until the waning moon tilted its eyebrow over the red rocks outside.

For a wedding gift I gave Jon a silver bear fetish like those worn by everyone in my family. While we were dancing, I saw a bright flash as it caught the light. Even my four-year-old nephew, B.J., my two-year-old niece, Cassy, and a few old Navajo grandmas were dancing that night. For a few moments my two parallel worlds combined.

Jon soon joined the New Mexico National Guard and enrolled in classes at the community college. Our life together had begun. Although many women physicians keep their maiden names, I decided to take Jon's last name. It was important to me that our family be connected and recognized by the same name. Moreover, I had never felt any real attachment to my maiden name, Cupp, especially since learning that Theron Cupp had not been related to me by blood. Since I was about to change my name, I also decided to take Grandma's maiden name, Arviso, as my own middle name. It was my Navajo family name, and I was proud to claim it. I was beginning a new life, and it seemed right to have a new name to enter it: so I changed my name legally to Lori Arviso Alvord.

The OR at GIMC had become so many things to me—professionally, culturally, and spiritually. It seemed fitting that I would also find a husband there. It was to be the place where I would find many of the most important things in my life.

Chapter Ten

▲▲▲▲

AT THE BIG
MEDICINE SPACE

The little Navajo girl with a neat French braid and brand-new high-top sneakers lay on her side on the examining table, her face glazed with pain. Her mother sat beside her. At the foot of the hospital bed stood her grandmother in full traditional dress—a bright cotton print skirt and a red velvet blouse with silver buttons, numerous squash blossom and beaded necklaces, and heavy silver-and-turquoise bracelets. She was wearing her most valuable belongings for this important visit to the city, all topped by a determined expression on her face.

It was a wet winter morning, and when my beeper had gone off in the predawn stillness, I looked up to see ice crystals making diamond patterns on the windows. Being married had many advantages. Companionship, commiseration, and help lifting heavy objects were a few of them. But it made answering late-night and early-morning calls much harder. I only reluctantly left the cozy bed where my sleeping husband was still curled up in blankets.

I dialed the pediatric ward's number and spoke to Dr. Prieto on the phone. "I have a little girl with abdominal pain,
especially in the right lower quadrant, a high white count,
and a fever," he said.

When I got to the hospital I was instantly thrust into
medical drama. The little girl was desperately in need of
help and the older generation was deeply afraid to agree
to it. Three generations of Navajo women stood before
me. Yet all decision-making power clearly belonged to the
grandmother.

The little girl's name was Melanie Begay, and while her
grandmother and mother watched anxiously I pressed my
hands against her warm skin. I felt the tenderness in her
belly that Dr. Prieto described. She winced noticeably, even
when I brushed gently against her. Her stomach felt tense,
like an inflated balloon. When I pressed down again, she began to cry. Tears pressed out of the corners of her eyes and
made coffee-colored stripes as they rolled down the sides of
her dusty face.

The look on her face was the look of a person who has
gone past discomfort to another country of suffering. In that
country the citizens are completely indifferent to what lies
around them. They neither notice things, hear speech, nor
see what is in front of them. The only language spoken is the
universal language of pain. All concentration is focused on
fighting it. I have seen my patients in this state many times,
and during my surgical residency, when I was so sick, my
own pain had demanded all my attention. In that condition
everything else ceases to exist.

Based on the result of the brief exam, as well as her high
white count and other preliminary evidence, I made an im-
mediate decision: Melanie should go right to the operating
room for an appendectomy. An "appy" is generally a routine
procedure, but some cases are critical. If the appendix is perforated, there is the possibility of infection and even death. I
did not know if little Melanie's appendix was perforated, but

it seemed very clearly to be infected. It could rupture at any moment.

Unfortunately Melanie's grandmother, Bernice Begay, overheard the Navajo nurses discussing Melanie's case earlier and immediately reacted. The *bilagáana* doctors were not going to cut open her granddaughter, she'd said loudly to a Navajo aide. Did we know for sure what was wrong inside her? There had to be something else we could do.

There is no single conclusive test for appendicitis. No blood test will give a positive identification of the condition. No X-ray has a 100 percent success rate for a diagnosis. An ultrasound procedure may suggest a problem, but it is inconsistent, and a CT scan may not only be inconsistent but may miss appendicitis altogether unless it is one of the newer "spiral CT scans," but we didn't have that at Gallop.

The truth is, surgeons become so accustomed to seeing patients with appendicitis that they can recognize it by clinical examination and intuition. Statistically, physicians are right about 80 percent of the time in diagnosing appendicitis in their female patients and 90 percent of the time in male patients. (The difference is due to the fact that gynecological problems may cause some confusion.) For children, there may be a dilemma between distinguishing appendicitis from intestinal infections.

As these thoughts raced through me, precious minutes were passing—and each one that passed made the situation more critical. What should I tell Melanie's grandmother—that I "felt" it was necessary to do this surgery? That I had a strong "intuition" that I should open up her granddaughter's body and take out a piece? I knew this was their worst nightmare.

I left the examining room to think about the best way to handle the situation. Maybe I could get through to the mother; maybe there were other relatives who could be called.

When I came back a few minutes later, I saw immediately

that Molly Begay, Melanie's mother, would be of no help to me in persuading Bernice. She looked tired, and was deferential to the older woman, as is customary in Navajo families. I should have known it: older women rule the roost in my world. They are honored, even revered. In many circumstances their words are tantamount to law. And the grandmother's jaw was set. She looked ready for a fight.

"*Yáat'ééh Shímásaní,*" I greeted her. *Hello, Grandmother.* She instantly looked up at me. I introduced myself in the Navajo tradition, telling her that I was from the *Tsi'naajinii* and *Ashįįhi Dineé* clans and was originally from Crownpoint. As we were talking, Roy Smith arrived and picked up where my Navajo left off. He and Bernice spoke congenially, and his presence seemed to comfort her. Sometimes I felt a little jealous of his easiness and the trust he instantly inspired in patients. But most of the time I just felt grateful.

My Navajo was improving with practice; the classes I'd taken had served me well. Frequently I understood the basic meaning of what my patients said, but rather than risk a mis-understanding, which in medicine could have grave conse-quences, I always asked an interpreter along when dealing with patients who did not speak English.

From Roy's questions I found out that Melanie had been having pain yesterday, that she'd not wanted dinner, and that her pain had gotten worse during the night. She had vomited several times. Roy said Bernice was very afraid of what we might do to her granddaughter. She did not want anyone to cut her.

Deep inside, I understood Bernice's fears. They came from the history of our people and our relationship to Anglo society. Bernice appeared to be in her seventies so I knew she'd had firsthand experience of Navajo land taken away, of children forcibly taken to white boarding schools, as had happened to my grandmother. At those schools their language and culture had been replaced by *bilagáana* beliefs. The American Bill of Rights had not applied to her until 1968. She had not the right to religious freedom until 1978.

She certainly remembered hearing about other historical events as well, like the Long Walk. In the spring of 1863, responding to the complaints of white settlers, who fought with the Navajos as the settlers moved into land held by the tribes, Colonel Kit Carson led a scorched-earth campaign that sent Navajo people fleeing to the mountains or to Canyon de Chelly. Carson took all the livestock and burned all the hogans and orchards. That winter the Navajo were starved into submission and eight thousand Navajo men, women, and children were forced to walk three hundred and fifty miles south to Bosque Redondo, near Fort Sumner, New Mexico.

The result was a disaster. The camp did not have enough supplies, and diseases like measles and smallpox were rampant. Medical care was deficient. The Navajos' desire to return to the canyonlands where they had grown corn and raised sheep for centuries was so strong that a Navajo leader in Fort Sumner told the army leaders: "What we want is to be sent back to our own country. Even if we starve there, we will have no complaints to make."[8]

Because of disease and starvation at Bosque Redondo, more than three thousand of my people never made it home. Every Navajo family has their own version of this story—based on the unique experiences of their own relatives. All three of my Navajo great-great-grandparents (both my grandmother's grandmothers and her Navajo grandfather) walked to Fort Sumner and back again. According to my grandmother, the soldiers treated them terribly, and when someone was tired or sick, they just pulled them out of line and made them sit under a tree in the shade until they could walk again. My maternal great-grandmother was just a teenage girl at the time.

"We were their prisoners. They made us walk all that way. The old ones, women and children too, while they rode their horses. Now they expect us to love white people," my grandmother had explained to me. "Isn't that crazy?"

The Long Walk to and from the prison camp in Fort Sumner is an event known to every Navajo man, woman, and child. Like the Holocaust for the Jews, it is the historical event that most illustrates our vulnerability as a race. I know that Bernice Begay was no exception: someone in her family had walked the long walk, too.

And she had no doubt heard that Navajo families were being forced to move again today, from the "joint use" land in Arizona that they have lived on for centuries and share with the Hopi. In 1974 the federal government passed a law calling for the land to be divided. Many Navajo people have called the ensuing government-enforced removal of people from the only homes they'd ever known "the second Long Walk."

Beyond historical events, stories and allegations have spread on the reservation about Native American women who were sterilized in Oklahoma in the 1950s as well as rumors that the Indian Health Service delivers substandard health care to Indian patients. While some of these stories are unfounded, it is true that IHS hospitals sometimes do not have the staffing or equipment that other hospitals consider necessary requirements. Even today, some of the doctors who work with the Navajo people are young and inexperienced: fresh out of their residencies or medical school, and staying for only a year or two to meet their medical school loan obligations.

My own personal experiences with the IHS as a Navajo and as a patient had been mixed. Growing up, we had agonizingly long waits whenever we went to see a doctor. But twice when my mother was very sick—once from the internal bleeding of an ectopic pregnancy and once from a miscarriage—she was successfully airlifted by the IHS from the reservation to a hospital in Albuquerque, where she was treated. I can still remember the deafening beat of the helicopter rotors when they came to get her. Had the IHS not reacted as efficiently as they did, she would have died.

In our years growing up in the reservation, little in our home lives could have prepared my sisters and me for as frightening an experience as being a patient at a modern hospital. Thrust into Melanie Begay's position—off the reservation, in a world of *bilagáana* strangers—we would have been completely out of our element, as today I felt sure she was. We would have been scared of the needles and the white-clad doctors and the unfamiliar surroundings. Coming from our childhood world of mesa games, the hospital would seem artificially lit and strange, the food peculiarly bland, the hospital equipment too shiny, alien, and intimidating.

Even though GIMC is a Navajo hospital, most of the physicians and nearly all the administrators are white. The chrome-and-steel-filled emergency room, where Melanie came in, is full of computer-operated machines and white curtained-off areas. In the words of Dr. Waxman, one of our OB-GYNs, "we have monitors to monitor the monitors." Nurses come every thirty minutes or so to check patients' vital signs.

But, in fact, Melanie was so sick, she noticed little around her. It was a good thing—I was sure she would have been terrified otherwise.

I was in a dilemma, too. I was supposed to represent the hospital, the medical establishment, the need to give prompt treatment. But my heart also engaged where only my brain and medical training were needed. A part of me was siding with this family.

I could see both sides of the story. One side—the trained

medical practitioner, who fathoms the body's mysteries as a detective directs a beam of light into a dark room to look for clues about the source of physical disharmony—said, *Roll her into the OR now!* But the Navajo part of me, who had once been a little girl, could see the inappropriateness of interfering. Navajo eyes warned: The beauty of the body would be disturbed. A surgical knife would defile an intact, miniature universe, with rules and systems that evolved naturally over millennia. I could see the sacredness of that body, how all its many parts are one harmonic system.

Melanie Begay's grandmother, refusing to let us operate, was shaping up as the perfect embodiment of my cultural conflict. I had suddenly been feeling it quite often recently. In my job I'd felt judged by others on the basis of race even though I was now a board-certified surgeon. "And how did you get into Stanford?" one colleague had asked me, insinuating that I was accepted only as a token. And in my marriage there were so many things I needed to explain to Jon. Navajo people feel many pressures when we marry outside our own. It is subtle, but it is strong, too. It is a veiled disapproval.

My Western medical training told me that the eight-year-old girl could die if we did not remove her appendix right away. But her grandmother's fears and objections were just as real and true. The two worlds were colliding. The solution lay somewhere in the uncharted territory between them. But at the moment, time was running out.

Probably the Begays had brought Melanie to GIMC, to *Azee Al'i Hotsaai'*, or "the big space where medicine is given," only as a last resort, after Navajo traditional medicine had been tried and she did not improve. I hoped I could find a way to explain to Bernice what we wished to do in a way that she could accept.

After much thought, I made my decision.

I told Bernice that the decision was hers to make. It

was something I had begun to tell patients more and more, a show of respect that I believed would be empowering; that they alone, not the doctors or anyone else, control the fate of their bodies. We doctors could not force them to do anything they did not wish to do. When I said this to Melanie's grandmother, she looked as though she weren't sure she could trust me. She seemed to be weighing whether I had another agenda.

In fact, she might be very upset soon, because the nurse informed me that some of the hospital social workers were seeking legal help to get a court order, so that surgery could be performed on the little girl in opposition to her family's desires. I did not want to bring in *bilagáana* authority—I believed the best solution lay in returning the power to Bernice.

Tim Simpson ran into me in the third-floor hallway and grabbed my elbow. "Everything going all right with the little girl?"

"They don't want the surgery," I said. "I'm doing my best to convince them."

"If you need any help, just call," he said reassuringly. I could see by his eyes that he saw the urgency of the situation and my own unwillingness to impose upon the family.

A few moments later, when I went back into the room, I explained to Bernice, " '*Ałkidáá'*, many years ago, *Shimásaní*, we did not have this surgery, and sometimes people who had what Melanie has, well, they didn't survive. But now, with a small operation to correct the problem, we can make her well again."

She looked at me. "You will let us decide the right thing for Melanie," she said.

"I will." I nodded and simultaneuslly wondered how.

When I'd given Bernice control of the situation, I'd prayed it would inspire her trust in me as a fellow Navajo as well as a surgeon and that she would come to the conclusion that surgery was the best option for Melanie.

But time was passing, and Bernice was still reticent. The social workers were making progress in obtaining the court order. Any second now, a brigade of hospital administrators would burst into the room and forcibly take Melanie into the OR. I would have to go with them, as their leader. I would have to betray this family and go with the people they saw as their opposition: the *bilagáana*.

Although the court order might save the girl's life, it could also be a cultural disaster, and it would make a liar and an enemy of me. To wrench Melanie from her family and take her to a place they did not want her to go could be extremely traumatic and frightening for her, and it would, in my view, increase the odds of complications during her surgery.

The family's relatives had been called in from around the reservation and while we waited for Bernice's decision, they began to arrive in the hospital room. On a bank of chairs, outside the room, a pile of well-worn jackets and wraps, cowboy hats and bags mounted. Chunks of snow and mud from boots melted into a brown soup around the door. The soft murmuring and clicking music of Navajo, from within, was accompanied by the sound of shuffling feet. For a while I stood helplessly waiting in the hall, wondering what exactly was being said.

I imagined Bernice telling the others that they must not allow us to do the surgery on Melanie. She might be saying that surgery is a *bilagáana* practice, but they are Navajos. She could raise the issue of the risk of surgery, which we had had to inform her about. Perhaps she was saying that they should take Melanie home and call the medicine men back. She might believe that the piece of Melanie that we extracted would fall into the wrong hands and someone would bewitch her. She might be saying that even the tiniest piece—a sliver of flesh or a hair—would do.

At nightfall Melanie's father, Victor Begay, arrived. He stood outside the room in the hallway, and from time to time other family members came out to speak with him. Because Melanie's grandmother, Victor's mother-in-law, was in the room, he was not allowed to enter. Among traditonal Navajos, mother-in-law avoidance is a strict cultural rule. He would not discuss even the crisis concerning his daughter with her.

A sense of fear had begun to emanate from the assembled family and from the individual members who emerged to speak with Victor in the hall. They had a look of growing intensity in their eyes.

Standing down the hall, I could see through a crack in the door that Melanie's grandmother was standing behind Melanie's mother, with her hand on her shoulder, while the mother bent over Melanie, caressing her head.

The little girl was moaning. It was a low, barely audible sound, more like a repeated whimper. A plastic doll snuggled beside her. Her fingers clutched its hair.

Soon it was dinnertime. The hospital staff slowly brought around bright stainless-steel carts filled with covered trays of food, like shiny steamships, making regular stops with their deliveries.

I was not on call and was about to drive home and have dinner with Grandma and Jon. But I told the nursing staff to beep me immediately if the Begay family came to a decision, and if they consented to it I would drive back and do the surgery.

Everyone on the floor knew the sensitivity of the situation. Outside the room a cluster of nurses had gathered, all of them wearing the same look of weighted anticipation. Victor, dressing in dusty cowboy boots, blue jeans, and a flannel shirt, looked like a man who just came in from a hard day's work. Just as I was heading off the floor, he indicated with a gesture of his head that he wished to speak with me. I went and stood beside him. I was on Navajo time now. Many minutes could pass before the time was right for us to speak of such personal things.

For a moment we were both silent, in a manner that indicates respect among Navajo people. We were careful not to look directly at each other. I broke the silence by greeting him.

"How is she doing, Doctor?" he asked, his eyes focused on the ground.

"Melanie is getting sicker," I said. "Her heart rate is going up, and so is her fever. She needs to have this operation before it's too late." I decided to push a little harder. "This is your decision—but if you decide against the surgery and Melanie doesn't make it, you may find your own decision very hard to live with."

My words hung between us in the air like a dark bird. If he listened to me, he would be going against the ancient Navajo ways, in which the women make decisions like these. He would be going against the will of his mother-in-law. For a very brief moment I let my eyes cross his face. His eyes, the color of dark stones, looked away.

A little while later, I was checking in one more time before heading out when my beeper went off.

Please tell me that she didn't rupture, I thought, and then allowed the worst-case scenario to flip through my mind: *Please tell me she isn't coding.* "Dr. Alvord, please call extension four-five-nine, four-five-nine," demanded the device at my hip.

I picked up the nearest phone and held my breath while it rang.

"Dr. Alvord?" asked the pediatrics nurse.

"Yes?"

Everything depended on the next few words I would hear. "The consent form has been signed."

Relief swept over me. I didn't know how the decision had been made or who had made it. I was just glad it had: we would operate on Melanie Begay, remove her infected appendix, and save her life.

Chapter Eleven

▲▲▲▲

"DO NOT TRY TO COUNT THE STARS"

One morning at dawn, First Man and First Woman saw a dark cloud over Gobernador Knob. Later they heard a baby cry. When they looked to see where the crying was coming from, they realized it came from within the cloud that covered the top of Gobernador Knob.

—NAVAJO HISTORY, PART I, CREATION

Don't look at bad things, Lori," Roy Smith cautioned me one morning, as we convened for rounds in the ICU. My friend warned me about becoming angry or getting stressed out. He'd gestured at the globe of my pregnant middle. "And be careful not to look at the bad parts of surgery."

I nodded with seriousness, willing to hear whatever pearls of wisdom he dispensed. I was still adjusting to pregnancy—I had not even realized I was pregnant until I was four months along. I'd thought I was missing a few periods as my body adjusted to discontinuing using the contraceptive Depo Provera. My colleagues—the nurses and doctors I worked with—had teased me about how as a doctor I am supposed to understand people's bodies, and yet I had missed all the clues with my own. Feeling sheepish, I had tried to compensate by becoming hyperaware—and by listening to all these Navajo wisdoms.

I soon learned that there were many things besides "looking at bad things" that I should be aware of. If I ate too much fatty food the baby would have trouble being born. If I saw an accident, it could hurt the baby. Above all, if I looked at a dead person, my baby would be sickly. I teased Jon about these, and the many things he was not supposed to do either. Jon laughed—he was delighted that we were having a baby. He had taken to rubbing my swollen belly and saying "Hi, wake up in there!"

Of all the warnings I heard, my favorite was the one about the stars. It said that if I counted them, I would have too many children. Staring up at the night sky, I wondered: Could I handle triplets? Twins?

But Roy's words stuck with me more than anyone else's. Maybe looking at "bad things" did have an adverse effect on pregnant women. Many traditional Navajos believe that just thinking bad thoughts can affect one's well-being. Maybe "not looking at bad things" was a way to stop a chain of bad thoughts from starting.

Western medicine too has begun to recognize the damaging effects of stress during pregnancy, and bad thoughts are certainly a source of stress. Research now shows that increased stress during pregnancy is associated with premature births. But Roy—with his long, graying hair pulled back into a ponytail and a sand-cast silver buckle at his waist—was telling me something he'd probaby heard from his grandmother. Once again Western medicine was "discovering" something that indigenous people had been aware of for hundreds, maybe even thousands of years.

Even before Roy mentioned it to me, though, I think I would have known it intuitively. Once I found out I was pregnant, I'd avoided watching violent television and movies. When Jon tuned in to a show with a lot of dead bodies and shoot-outs, I left the living room, as though looking at it could open a door for the violence to enter the warm sea inside me, where my baby was floating peacefully.

I also tried to avoid confrontations and arguments. But with surgery it was more difficult: how could I avoid seeing trauma? I'd been doing my best to steer clear of difficult cases, but it isn't always clear from the start which ones those will be.

The whole pregnancy, as I said, had been a delightful surprise. I had not planned on getting pregnant so soon after marriage. I was busy with my surgical practice, setting up a home with Jon, taking care of Grandma, and giving talks and seminars at Navajo high schools. Recently I had been asked by the NIH Office of Research in Women's Health to serve on the national task force for the recruitment and retention of women in clinical studies. The purpose of the task force was to address the problem of underrepresentation and even exlusion of women from important health studies. We listened to people from the scientific and lay communities, made recommendations, and developed a report recommending needed changes. On various occasions I had to fly to Washington to attend meetings and panels and testify. In short, it was not a time I would have chosen to get pregnant, but I had to ask myself: Would there ever be a time I would think was ideal? I thought not. My pregnancy seemed to have been decided by some force in the universe larger than myself. I was thirty-six. I would not have chosen it right then, but it had chosen me.

I found out when I traveled to Washington, D.C., for a thoracoscopy course. While lying on the bed at Sue's mother's house, where I was staying, I palpated my abdomen, thinking it felt slightly bloated. Suddenly my fingers, so used to feeling the abdomens of my patients, came across a new shape: I thought I could feel the top of my uterus!

When I got home, I took a home pregnancy test, and when it came out positive, I called Robyn Molsberry—"Mols," Tim Simpson's wife (and an OB-GYN surgeon)—and made an appointment. "I think I can feel my uterus," I told her. "No way," she'd replied, "you'd have to be quite far along to feel it." She'd been right about that.

As my pregnancy advanced, I wondered what "bad things" I might have already seen and if they were somehow affecting the baby. There had been a three-year-old with an infected foot that wouldn't heal right, a nineteen-year-old motor vehicle accident victim, and a quadriplegic on a ventilator who had developed diabetes and needed insulin.

In the wake of Roy's warning, I began to notice all the suffering, pain, and death I regularly saw: patients who spent day after day in the ICU. I realized that I had become a bit numb and I wondered if the abdominal pain that I was feeling was a result of the disharmony that I couldn't keep out of my life.

Then Roy and one of the Navajo nurses mentioned it: if my pelvic pain kept up, perhaps I should consider seeing a medicine man. But I found myself thinking things weren't *that* bad.

Despite words of consolation from doctors and sisters, however, pelvic pain continued to trouble me. I was even afraid I could lose my baby from it. Perhaps it sounds superstitious to a *bilagáana* consciousness, but sometimes it felt like the universe was drifting off course and that forces I did not know about were gripping my life. I was afraid there was something wrong with my pregnancy, that somehow I was out of sync with the forces of fertility and maternity.

One morning when I went into the clinic, someone had found a newborn baby left in a bathroom at the hospital. I heard the nurses talking about it and was terribly upset. How could the mother leave him? I shook with rage. But I cautioned myself not to get upset, and began to seriously consider seeing a medicine man.

Are such bursts of disharmony in our lives symptomatic of larger, more endemic, global imbalances? Navajo philosophy—in which everything in the universe is of equal importance, from a tiny blue-tailed lizard to a herd of deer to a population of humans to a meteor shower—would suggest that the appearance of small problems is a symptom of something larger. My abdominal pains and the abandoned infant seemed to be parts of a larger issue. Maybe a *hataałii* could correct this imbalance or my body's reaction to it.

Some doctors seem to have disharmony in their practices. *Some* surgeons often come across major difficulties in the OR. They are collectively referred to as "black clouds." Such doctors always seem to attract "problem" patients, with endless complications in their cases. They are like magnets for medical disaster. Once they are singled out and recognized as black clouds, they are often teased by the medical staff. Having one on call with you is tantamount to sending out an advertisement saying: "Come one, come all—we're having a special on really sick surgery patients." Their black-cloud status is a joke, in part, but there is also something serious about it. It is not that they are bad doctors. It is more that they are plagued by constant medical bad luck. If they were Navajo, they would be sent for a ceremony to restore their world to harmony.

I was not a black cloud, but I was beginning to feel disharmony in my life. So when I went in for my next prenatal checkup, I was pleased that I could tell my doctor that I'd not had another episode of pelvic pain. That optimism faded fast when Claire, an OB-GYN on staff, gave me the bad news: my blood pressure was up to 130 over 80.

"This is not good, Lori," she said. "It looks like you definitely have PIH."

I sighed. It was pregnancy-induced hypertension, also known as preeclampsia. "So what happens now?"

"What happens is you go home, you lie down, and you stay put. I mean it, or we'll have to hospitalize you." Then she added: "This means no more surgery."

"Okay, okay," I said. "I promise."

I checked on a few patients on my way out and went home. But once there I could not sit still. I paged through a few medical texts to find out more about PIH. Apparently it is quite common, but it can be serious. If the blood pressure keeps climbing it can signal disaster—seizures and even comas.

Just a few days before, I'd been a healthy, happy expectant mother–surgeon, having her baby shower at Sue and Joe's new house. My colleagues from the hospital, Grandma, Jon, and even the woman who gave me flute lessons, Randy Whitman, had all come out to a barbecue on the back porch overlooking mesas and the distant red rocks of the reservation. They'd brought gifts of all sorts from tiny Pendleton blankets (loved by Navajos) and moccasins to cradleboards and mobiles. Now all of the sudden I was on bedrest and threatened with hospitalization and seizures. For the first time in a long time, I found myself home with no chance of a beeper going off.

"Just lying down" was really hard for me. I'd flip through the TV channels, surfing through talk shows, old movies, and news, perhaps watching a little here or there about Women Who Dress Too Sexy and Teens Who Think Their Mothers Are Too Pretty. I tried to get into a book but I read the same page of *Return of the Native* twenty times. The only nice thing about being on bedrest was that Grandma liked having someone around all day.

The weekend went by like that—rental movies, Chinese takeout from Gallup's one passable Chinese restaurant, and writing and reading in a semireclining position on the living room couch. Jon spent a lot of time working on a white cedar cradle in the garage. And although a peaceful, domestic feeling filled the house, I was feeling somewhat restless and bored.

On Monday, when I went back to the hospital, my blood pressure was down a little but still too high. The OB-GYN nurse strapped the white Velcro of the fetal monitor around my melon-shaped belly, and I listened to the *blub-blub* sound of the baby for a while.

"He's doing just fine," they said. It was me they were worried about.

"We'll give you another week, Lori, and if your blood pressure doesn't go down, we'll have to induce." The baby wasn't due until August 29, and it was only the first week of August.

All right, I'd said to myself. So it's not the way I've envisioned birthing. I'd wanted a traditional Navajo-style birth, or at least something like it. But frankly, I was beginning to think any birth at all would be a huge relief. I felt swollen all over and nervous about the hypertension. Induction wouldn't be so bad, I decided.

But first I'd made up my mind to do one more thing.

I wouldn't enlighten my doctors about it right away, since they had threatened to hospitalize me if I didn't take the bedrest order seriously, but I was going to take a trip.

A quick trip over to Tuba City, Arizona.

I'd been thinking about it for weeks. It was as much for my baby as for me. With just a few phone calls and a little research, I had found him. While I had wanted to develop a relationship with a medicine man, I never imagined it would be one where I would be the patient. Like my patients before me, I was going to see a *hataałii*.

▲▲▲▲

Chapter Twelve

THE SPIRIT
HORSE'S BRIDLE

With beauty before me, there may I walk.
With beauty behind me, there may I walk.
With beauty above me, there may I walk.
With beauty below me, there may I walk.
With beauty all around me, there may I walk.
In beauty it is finished.

—BLESSING WAY

To get to Tuba City from Gallup, you drive through the tall pine-forested hills above Windowrock and then descend into the naked, many-layered canyonlands of Arizona. It is a three-and-a-half-hour trip through two worlds—from hogan-dotted Dinetah to the stark, sacred mesas of the Hopi, where HUD villages cluster on empty plateaus.

The morning I went to Tuba City, Grandma was walking down from the hogback cliff. When she got to the front door and saw me in the driveway, I told her I was going. She turned her gaze toward me, her eight-months-pregnant granddaughter, and said, "Don't hit any bumps."

A few hours later, as I passed through the choppier patches of the two-lane highway, I thought of her words. I was so big, it was a snug fit beneath the steering wheel of our new Four-Runner, which had seemed so roomy a few months earlier, when we bought it with our expanding family in mind.

While driving it through the winding hills of Gallup's Boardman Road, Robyn had come upon the perfect name for the baby. We wanted to have a name with meaning, and I wanted the name to be associated with the bear spirit. We would name him Kodiak—for the great black Alaskan bear. We could call him Kodi for short.

This journey, driving hundreds of miles west against all common sense when I had been ordered on bedrest for hypertension that threatened seizures and worse, might turn out to be a colossal error in judgment. But something told me Kodi and I needed to do this, and that it was the best thing I could do for us.

By noon, when I stopped near Keam's Canyon for a soda, it was well over a hundred degrees. The sun beat down on the pavement by the gas station, softening the asphalt. Little drops of sweat glistened on my forehead in the rearview mirror. Inside the gas station I caught a glimpse of my reflection in a refrigerator case. Who was this enormous woman, driving into the middle of nowhere on one of the hottest days of the year? In some cultures this act could be considered certifiable insanity. I did a double take. I suppose it's like this for all very pregnant women—I hardly recognized myself.

I drove on through vast stretches of desert land, with horizons that stretched for miles. Some of the land I passed was reclaimed Navajo land, and a few enclaves of Navajos along this route had resisted the relocation. I'd seen their photographs—ancient Navajo *shimasánís* and *shínális,* standing outside their hogans with twelve-gauge shotguns.

Weeks before my blood pressure shot up, when the problems in my pregnancy first began, I'd been thinking about this trip. But years ago, when I was in medical school, I'd already dreamed of meeting a traditional person who could teach me more about my tribe's own medicine. Yet it goes against Navajo convention to approach a medicine man and ask to be taught. Such students are chosen, just as medicine men are chosen or spiritually guided, usually when they are very young.

Now I needed help. Although I knew I was going to Tuba City as a patient, a part of me was excited to be encountering Navajo medicine. Perhaps this man could help me become more of a better healer in my own practice.

The right person had crossed my path. His name was even *hataałii*—Thomas Hataathlii. In addition to performing the Beauty Way ceremony, he was a counselor at the Tuba City IHS hospital. His picture was in *Tribal College* magazine—a special issue on Native Americans in medicine. He was an intelligent-looking man with glasses, looking right out of the picture, like a person staring out a window. Unbelievably, there was even a Dartmouth connection—for the past few years he'd sponsored workshops for Dartmouth Native American students, often far from home and alienated at the exclusive eastern school. He'd take them on camping trips, build sweat lodges with them, and try to instill a feeling of belonging that would make it easier for them to stay in school. When Dartmouth got its new Native American House on campus, the old Occum Inn, it was Thomas who performed the house blessing. When we spoke on the phone, he told me he knew of me, and had heard of my work as a surgeon at Gallup Indian Medical Center.

In some ways our lives were similar, both trying to live in the bureaucratic, Anglo world of the IHS, our employer, and the Navajo world. In the Navajo world he was so revered that at mealtimes the elder people walked behind him and waited until he'd tell them to eat. In his other world, at the IHS, people might casually ask him to get them a cup of coffee.

He was a combination of a young medical professional (he worked as a counselor and therapist) and a keeper of traditional Navajo ways. His sense of humor and spirit, his emodiment of my own duality, his wisdom at such a young age, and his balanced approach to life were evidence that I was right in my instincts to drive to Tuba City.

I arrived late for our appointment and drove through the small BIA town quickly, noticing how closely it resembled Crownpoint. Clusters of tall trees and grassy squares surrounded old stone buildings in the middle of the dusty desert, and twenty-four-hour gas stations with little supermarkets attached stood sentry. There was not much else. Dusty pickups passed me on either side. Signs pointed the way to the hospital.

The glass-framed directory in the hospital entranceway spoke volumes about the community. The problems of a conquered people were inscribed here:

Mental Health
TB Control
Dialysis
Fetal Alcohol Syndrome

I knew the IHS statistics well enough. Indian people served by the IHS have a 438 percent greater chance of alcoholism, a 400 percent greater chance of tuberculosis, a 155 percent greater chance of diabetes, and a 131 percent greater chance of motor vehicle accident than the general U.S. population. Native people are the poorest ethnic group in the country, five times more likely than anyone else to live without plumbing, and they are now in danger of losing vital government funding—funding awarded through a series of complicated treaties—as a result of drastic proposed budget cuts. But reneged treaties are nothing new. Ours has always been and still remain a population at risk.

I followed the arrow to Mental Health and there found Thomas's office. I sat on a bench outside. After a few minutes a man emerged and signaled to me. "Lori?"

"Hi," I said.

"I was wondering how you were going to make it down here by noon from Gallup."

I smiled sheepishly. "I forgot how far it is."

In person the tall, thin man with a roundish face and a beautiful bracelet, ring, and belt buckle studded with turquoise looked amazingly young. We tend to think of medicine men as older, leathery, and timeworn, with faces canyoned with lines and crow's-feet. Here was a handsome, athletic-looking man probably not much older than myself—maybe even younger.

When I walked into his office, the first thing I saw was the Dartmouth coffee mug on his desk. He explained that his supervisor, the director of mental health at the Tuba City IHS hospital, psychiatrist Elise Egerter, was Dartmouth-educated and had taken him to Dartmouth to meet the Native American students there.

For about half an hour we spoke in the Navajo style of communication, drawing verbal circles around each other. Nothing direct, at first, nothing too personal. But as I sat there taking Thomas in, I began to get a sense of who he was, and I felt he was getting a sense of me.

We began, as always, by revealing our relations and clans. He named his and I named my own, and then we moved on to discuss friends of our families and friends of our families' friends, until we finally discovered all the places where our lives intersect. This isn't so hard in a nation as small as ours. Before long one usually discovers that one's cousin's husband was someone's else's volleyball coach in high school, or some such thing. Thomas and I were related by clan—the *Ashįįhi Dineé*, his main clan, is also the clan of my father's real father, Dan Showalter. All of this talk—the informal formalities—was necessary before I could get down to the reason I had come to see him.

His office, a small, warm room with a cozy couch and a culttered-looking desk, was filled with pictures of his two little daughters and others of himself, running.

"When I was four years old," he said, "my grandfather told me to run every morning toward the dawn, so I did. And I've been running ever since." I nodded. It is a tradition to run to the east at dawn to greet Dawn Boy, one of the Navajo holy people. Many people bow toward the new dawn, and toss a pinch of corn pollen over their shoulder. But Thomas had taken the running to a whole new level. His office pictures showed him running in marathons and crossing finish lines with a big number pinned to his shirt.

Thomas grew up taking care of his uncle's livestock near an area called Coal Mine, where his grandfather, Ned Hataathlii, a well-known medicine man, once lived. As a small child, not long after he'd begun running, he had an experience there that forecast the rest of his life.

"One morning when I was herding sheep, I found a place where many sticks littered the ground, partially obscuring an old bridle. I picked it up and used it to tie up the sheepdog. Later, on my way home, I threw it away.

"The next morning, as usual, we went running at dawn. My two brothers were about fifty yards ahead of me, and when we were not far from the place I'd found the old bridle, I saw a horse running fast toward me. It didn't make any sound. I panicked and ran away from it, and my brothers tried to catch up with me. When I turned around to see where they were, that horse was gone.

"My grandfather told me, 'Where those sticks were coming up, when you took that bridle, you touched the things of another one who lived there. That horse was a spirit horse.'"

When that person had died, the grandfather told Thomas, his hogan was destroyed and his horse was killed so he could ride it in the spirit world. "You touched the spirit world," said Thomas's grandfather.

Ever since that day, Thomas told me, his family knew he would follow a spiritual path. When he finished high school and was about to go to college, his mother cautioned him.

"Don't go, Thomas," she said. "Speaking English so much will change your words." As he told me this, his long fingers brushed across the part of his throat where his voicebox was.

Speaking Navajo has many levels, and deeper ways of communicating than speech alone. I was acquainted with only the most rudimentary aspects, but others can hear subtleties of meaning in every sound. It is both a tonal and a glottal language, which means that every slight inflection, every noise that may sound to an outsider like a clearing of the throat, has meaning. Some elder Navajos are famous just for their speaking ability. Thomas asked me if I could speak our language. I told him I was learning. "I understand more than I can speak," I said.

Then he told me his family believed that he had the right sounds for songs. "My parents and grandparents knew about my memory, and about my spirit, and they knew that I was the one out of the family who could be the next medicine man. My father had tried, but he couldn't remember the songs. So I didn't go to college. I didn't want to lose the way of speaking."

One day Thomas's grandfather gave him a mountain soil medicine bundle, containing soil from each of the four sacred mountains. Then he began his training. At the time when I met him in 1995, he was one of the youngest, if not the youngest, Navajo medicine man. He performed the Blessing Way ceremony—more than three hundred songs— and had learned parts of the nine-day Night Way ceremony. He had done Blessing Ways all over the reservation and had even been asked to perform one in Canada, for the people there who also call themselves the *Diné*. They are a part of the Athabascan language group—the same group to which the Navajo language belongs. Many people believe they are the ancestors of the Navajo.

"I learned the ceremonies by staying up all night sixteen times a year, not by tape-recording them," Thomas said. "My grandfather told me to do it this way. 'Make the effort,' he told me. 'You are gifted.' "

After he learned some of the ceremonies, he finally did go away to school—to Northern Arizona University—where he studied on a track scholarship. But he came home often and kept learning the ceremonies.

His stories about his grandfather reminded me of Grandma and her wry sense of humor and irony. When Neil Armstrong walked on the moon, Thomas told his grandfather about it.

"Grandfather, the white men went to the moon," he said, and pointed up in the middle of the sky, where the moon hung like an ornament in a tree.

"They went too far, then," his grandfather replied. "They should have met it when it first came up." He pointed at the horizon. "Down here. That would have been closer."

Thomas and I spoke for a few hours in his office, and he went over many things with me, describing all the major and minor ceremonies, some of which he could perform. I spoke to him about the fact that I'd never had a *kinaałdá,* and how I thought it might have prevented later problems in my life. He listened intently.

He then spoke to me about the four sacred mountains and explained that the air we breathe today existed long ago, when the world was just darkness. Each of the four directions, he said, represented a different part of the day. East, where Blanco Peak is, is dawn; south, where Mount Taylor is, is twilight; west and San Francisco Peak is yellow evening; and north, where La Plata Peak is, is folding darkness.

I had heard these things all my life, but no one had ever sat down with me and gone over them in such detail, with such care. Bits and pieces of it were familiar, but Thomas connected them all together. He gave me the string to tie all my knowledge together in a pattern, like a rug.

Sitting in front of his desk, with one ankle pulled over a knee, he said: "I have performed traveling songs for many young Navajos who are going away to college and returning-home songs for veterans of Desert Storm." Then he said, "Lori, I have also sung songs for women having trouble during pregnancy and women about to give birth."

Usually, he said, traditional women who are about to give birth have a ceremony in their eighth month. On Friday night an upbringing prayer is performed and a sacred mountain prayer; on Saturday morning, sacred footprints and a cleansing or bathing prayer are sung; and starting on Saturday evening a whole night of chanting is performed. For four days the woman cannot cut meat, have an angry outburst, dig, take a shower, have a haircut, or have sexual activity.

Then Thomas asked me, "What is it that brought you here?"

I did not know quite what to say. I had not known what to expect from him, but he had exceeded all my hopes. A part of me felt that he was testing me, as Lujan used to do. A part of me thought he already knew that I was having problems with my pregnancy. Briefly I told him about my rising blood pressure, and the threat of seizures. "I want to do what is best for the baby," I said. "Some of the nurses told me to find a medicine man."

"How much Navajo can you understand?" he asked. "Do you know what *hózhǫ́ne háaz'dlíí* means?"

I nodded. " 'It is beautiful all around me.' "

Then he told me he would do a prayer for me and my baby. "It starts from the east, then goes to the south, west, and north," he said, and asked me to repeat these words after him: *'Ashchí,* "to give birth."

And again, *hózhǫ́ne háaz'dlíí,* "It is beautiful all around me."

"Pray for the baby," he said. "Have you brought any blankets or turquoise to pay me for the ceremony?" he asked. I shook my head, embarrassed. As we left the hospital to drive to his home, where he kept his grandfather's mountain soil bundle, I berated myself. Why hadn't I remembered to ask him on the phone what I should bring? I remembered well the piles of deer hides and jewelry my family had brought to medicine men. But I had heard that sometimes medicine men accept cash instead. I wrote out a check, hoping it would suffice as payment.

One might imagine a medicine man's home as a traditional hogan, out somewhere on a deserted mesa, but this was the 1990s, and Thomas Hataathlii lived in a new trailer park in Tuba City. I followed his white pickup to the park, not far from the hospital, where brand-new trailers and pickups were lined up in a neat row against the blue sky.

Outside his double-wide trailer, two neon orange-and-pink children's bicycles lay by the door, with all the earmarks of the rush of children hurrying into their home. Inside, everything was neat and tidy and modern.

On one wall were studio photographs of Thomas and his wife and their two daughters and an adjacent wall was covered with the medals and ribbons he'd won in marathons. In 1979 he'd placed first in a ten-kilometer run in Page, Arizona. He had another first-place plaque for a 1993 10K run at Lake Powell, and a third-place plaque for a 1993 run at Colorado Belle Dam River. These were but a few of many. Across from the couch, above the television, was a small village of trophies—all for the running his grandfather had taught him to do each morning, to greet the dawn and the new sun rising in the east.

Thomas explained that his wife and daughters had gone to Flagstaff for the day to visit some of their in-laws. Then he pushed back the couch and coffee table and made a space in the middle of the floor. He unrolled a Pendleton blanket onto the carpet and put two pillows down on top of it. Signaling me to sit down on one of the pillows, he went into the bedroom.

He returned with a blue sash, which he proceeded to tie around his head. Suddenly Thomas Hataathlii *looked* like a medicine man.

He'd also brought out several bundles of cloth, which he unrolled to reveal beautiful eagle feathers, tied together with a strip of leather, and a small leather pouch. It was his grandfather's medicine bundle.

Instructing me to kneel on the blanket, Thomas placed the feathers and the medicine bundle in my hands. Then, sitting by my side, he began to sing the prayer for my baby.

His voice was the breathy, glottal music of Navajo, and with each phrase of the music, his body rocked a tiny bit forward and back again. It was the voice his mother had warned him not to ruin by "speaking English so much."

> *"Hózhǫ́ne háaz'dlíi,*
> *hózhǫ́ne háaz'dlíi,*
> *hózhǫ́ne háaz'dlíi,*
> *hózhǫ́ne háaz'dlíi."*

He showed me how to hold the medicine bundle and the feathers in front of my chest and then pull them toward my heart four times while we chanted the words. His chants surrounded me in a steady rhythm as I repeated,

> "It is beautiful all around me."

Then he showed me how to press the bundle and feathers against the four corners of my body. I had to sit in a position nearly impossible for an eight-months-pregnant woman, with my legs straight out in front of me. "Now I am going to do the earth prayer," he said, going to the sink to wash his hands.

When he came back, he sat beside me on the floor and

began to sing again, this time with his eyes shut. It was almost as if he had entered a trance. I shut my eyes, too, and let his voice enter me. For what seemed like a long time, he sang. I recognized some of the words, passing through me. And when I heard him sing *'ashchí,* and *hózhǫ́ne háaz'dlíí,* I whispered along.

The songs passed over me, around me, and through me. Beauty was above me, below me, behind me, in front of me. It felt like a cool breeze.

In a little while he stood up and extracted from his medicine bundle a pinch of corn pollen, which he sprinkled over me, touching points on my body gently, staining them bright yellow: my ankles, knees, shoulders, face, and head. Then he sprinkled it in a line over all of me and in a circle around me and placed a little on my tougue.

Next he sprinkled a little bit of the pollen onto the floor and then tied up his mountain bundle again.

"Now go outside, Lori, and turn around once, and then come back in."

I opened the door and walked out onto the wooden steps outside the trailer. The heat of the day was intense. It felt as if I'd opened an oven. I turned around once and came back inside. The ceremony was ended.

There was so much I wanted to say. I wanted to ask him to come to GIMC and speak to the staff, I wanted to accompany him to the Blessing Way in Canada, and I wanted to find out when he was going back to Dartmouth. But all of this seemed out of place, in light of what had just happened. It could wait until another time.

"Thank you so much, Thomas," I said. "This means a great deal to me."

"You are welcome, Lori," he said. "Keep in touch."

I pressed the check into his hand as I headed toward the door and the inferno of the Tuba City afternoon.

As I stepped down into the dirt yard I thought I heard him say one last thing, almost under his breath: "Be humble." I wondered when I would see him again.

Even though it was probably a hundred degrees or more, I felt calm, peaceful, and happy as I drove off. I hardly even considered the long drive ahead of me.

It was late afternoon, and clouds were building in the south. Great thunderheads massed in gray piles like uncarded wool.

The trip home went so fast, I scarcely noticed it. Somewhere along the way, as the Four-Runner dipped down into the sheep meadows and box canyons of Arizona, I realized that I felt happy, and I knew that everything would somehow be all right for Kodi and me and Jon.

As I approached the wooded hills outside Windowrock, I could see the precise place where I would leave the baking sun and enter the storm. A silver-gray curtain of rain pulled across the world before me in Dinetah. The cars driving toward me had their lights on and were covered with shiny drops of water. In the back of the storm a few crooked javelins of lightning flashed. And then to my right the hazy arc of a broken rainbow touched its purple-and-gold foot down in a meadow that seemed mere feet away from the highway.

"We're almost home, Kodi," I said.

▲▲▲▲

We'd had an argument between us for weeks, Jon and I. He wanted to give out cigars when Kodi was born. I didn't.

"They're stinky, and they cause cancer," I complained whenever the subject came up.

"It's a tradition," he retorted.

"Whose tradition? It isn't my tradition. Navajos don't traditionally give out cigars."

"Then you can hand out corn pollen or something," he said.

"We don't 'hand out corn pollen' when a baby is born!"

He always joked about Navajos giving out corn pollen for

every special occasion. He knew it drove me crazy. In the end we agreed that he could hand out a few cigars if he wanted. I bought him a box—pink bubblegum cigars.

When I got home from Tuba City, he greeted me at the door with a kiss. "Thomas did a prayer for me and Kodi," I said.

"That's good." He rubbed the globe of my belly with his hands. Then he put his finger up to my forehead, and when he brought it down, it was stained bright yellow. "Aha! Corn pollen!" he said.

Chapter Thirteen

▲▲▲▲

A KNOTTED SASH

*With the rainbow hanging high over
your head,
Come to us soaring.*

—PRAYER FROM THE NIGHT CHANT

A very special custom occurs after a Navajo baby is born: a celebration of the baby's first laugh. The soul (also called "the wind") enters the body soon after birth. A baby's laugh is a sign that the soul has become attached to the body.

When a baby laughs for the first time, the person who made the baby laugh must host a party. They buy candy for the guests, and during the celebration small pieces of rock salt are placed in a woven basket. The baby "gives" pieces of salt to each of the guests. Then the guests are given the candy. It is believed that by doing this, the baby will grow up to be generous and giving.

I thought ahead to the great laugh party Kodi would have, to distract myself from the unpleasant, real situation at hand. In spite of weeks of bedrest and temporarily quitting surgery, my blood pressure did not go down. When I came in for my checkup with Mols, it was 144 over 88. This is the danger zone for an expectant mom, and my pressure was rising, not falling.

So on a Monday morning, Jon and I gathered my necessities and packed them in two small duffel bags, including my favorite fuzzy red-and-yellow blanket, and we drove to GIMC. The decision had been made: They were going to induce labor. Because I was an enrolled tribal member, I could be a patient at GIMC—something most of my colleagues couldn't be. It meant that I would soon be in a complete role reversal—the faces that were usually at my side, listening to my advice, would be hovering over me, consulting with one another about my condition.

From time to time every doctor thinks about moments like this. We are all aware that our own bodies are susceptible to the same fates as our patients'. Illness can be pretty scary for us, since we know much too much to be altogether comfortable.

"It's like, damn, you *are* the patient," Mols explained the feeling from her own recent delivery. It was hard to imagine Robyn relinquishing her role as baby doctor to become a baby doctor's patient.

But I decided to make the best of it. Weeks ago, I'd alerted all my favorite anesthesiologists and asked them to be on hand to do my epidural.

My experience with patients like Evelyn Bitsui had showed me that difficult patients are the ones who experience complications, so I was determined not to be difficult. I would be the most compliant, most easygoing, happiest patient the place had ever seen. I had been working hard to control my episodes of anger and impatience, especially in the OR, with a lot of success. Now, while I was under the most stress and discomfort I would probably ever feel in my life, I had to control any urges I had to yell.

In fact, I felt pretty happy, even though a few hours after my arrival, my arm was already bruising blue from missed efforts at finding a good vein for the IV heplock. Everyone on staff had given it a go, even Sue, and Jon was told he couldn't try because if *he* missed, I'd be mad at him. They'd finally had to call the ER to get our pro, Cal Marshall, a giant of a man with a giant heart to match—he'd taken good care of Grandma one night in the ER when she'd had chest pains.

"Everybody out of the room," Cal demanded, then expertly felt the obscured and tentative blood vessels in my hands and the backs of my wrists. Many of them had been blown from my episode in the hospital at Stanford. He caught and punctured one, slipping in the needle with ease. He'd needed quiet and privacy to do the job right, he said, as in catching a fish.

The white Velcro straps of the fetal monitors had been strapped around my middle, registering Kodi's heart rate and movement, and with the IV finally in, I lay on my back, playing with Kodi's foot with one finger, moving it back and forth. Either Dr. Claire Wendland or Dr. Alan Waxman would be delivering Kodi. I trusted them both.

"But I'm going to catch him," Jon said. "My little blond boy."

Weeks ago, I had heard Mom and Jon laughing in the kitchen. "Wha-aat?" I called from the living room.

"Oh, your mom just said, 'Won't she just die if the baby turns out to be blond?'" said Jon.

They found this funny because they were the two blonds in the family, and I sensed a conspiracy between them to increase their numbers. It was also an opportunity to poke fun at me, the most "pro-Indian" member of the family. When I was a teenager I'd resented the fact that I was part white. Later I realized that my attitude had caused my mother, the woman I loved the most in my life, a great deal of unnecessary pain. Perhaps it would be poetic justice if my husband and child were both blond.

"Don't get your hopes up too high," I said to Jon now, as I lay on my back. I warned him about the low odds that Kodi would be blond and the decreasing odds that he'd be able to deliver him. "We may have to go C-section."

In my dream delivery, Jon *would* have caught Kodi. I

would also integrate all sorts of traditional Navajo ways into the birth. But due to my dangerously high blood pressure, this baby needed to come out soon—and by state-of-the-art high-tech means. I would have to forgo my imagined traditional birth for medical pragmatism.

When a Navajo woman gives birth, many rituals are carefully followed. For example, at the first signs of labor, cedar is smudged, and the woody, sweet smell of burning purifies the air. The cedar smoke is used to induce serenity and good thoughts in the mother. Also, a red-and-white woven sash, prepared with corn pollen, is hung from the ceiling of the hogan. The mother-to-be either squats or stands over a trough that has been dug in the hogan floor and spread with warm sand or a sheepskin. The sheepskin is a good surface for the woman to kneel on during labor and it also works well for catching the afterbirth. Holding on to the sash, the mother-to-be pulls with the spasms of labor. This is thought to help ease the pains of delivery, and good thoughts are to flow into her from the sash. Amusingly, Western medicine is only now realizing the benefits of labor in a vertical sitting or squatting position. Such a position lends gravity's assistance to the delivery, and allowing the woman to put her feet on the floor can create more effective pushing during labor.

A few other Navajo traditions were interesting to me. For one, Navajos are very careful not to touch the placenta, amniotic fluid, or blood of childbirth. It is felt to be very powerful and could possibly hurt those who come in contact with it.

Before the labor, also, the mother is given an herbal tea drink. Ironically, some say those drinks hasten labor, much like the medications given by the OB-GYN staff.

During labor a medicine man might brush the woman's kneeling body with an eagle feather, or unravel a rope prepared with slipknots over her abdomen, while chanting songs from the Blessing Way. If the labor takes a long time, the medicine man might ask the family to untie any knots in their possessions, such as knots on ropes tying up horses or other livestock. It is believed that untying knots will prevent the baby from getting tangled in the umbilical cord.

I'd wanted to add at least a few of the rituals in my baby's delivery. I'd brought along a Navajo sash, and I'd looked all over the delivery room for a place to hang it, but there was no place on the ceiling to tie it. The nurses told me that other Navajo women had simply tied the sash onto the end of the bed and pulled on it lying down.

In a traditional birth the entire family stays in the hogan with the mother-to-be—even grandparents and little children. After the baby is born, the placenta and umbilical cord are taken, by either the mother or grandmother, and saved. They are placed with the dead skin from the umbilicus. Later, they are buried in a special place—a place that symbolizes their hopes for the child. A child that the parents want to become a horseman will have his placenta buried by a corral; a child who is hoped to become an excellent weaver will have its placenta buried by the south side of the hogan, where the weaving loom is located.

Once I teased my mother, "You must have left my placenta right in the hospital," I said, "and that's why I became a doctor."

"You're right," she said with a laugh. "I did."

Many years ago my mother told me the story of my birth, in a military hospital in Tacoma, Washington, where my father was stationed in the army. A few weeks before Christmas thirty-seven years ago, my father, mother, and I had scared the nursing staff half to death. Another baby was born in the same maternity ward on the same day I was born. She was a blond, pink-skinned baby girl, born to a Japanese woman. I was a dark-skinned baby with a hint of oriental features—wide cheeks and almond-shaped eyes—also characteristic of the Navajo. When the nurses saw me in my blond mother's arms, they thought the babies might have been given to the wrong mothers. They'd whispered nervously in the hall, not sure what to do or how to approach the two women. That evening two men arrived on the ward—a tall blond man and an Asian-looking one. The nurses gathered around to see what the fathers would make of the complexions of their new daughters. But then the blond man went into the room with the Japanese woman, and my Navajo father went into the room with my mother. There was a burst of laughter from the nurses when they finally figured it out.

A lot of variations on the theme of childbirth might occur for me the next day, but one thing was for sure: none of the nurses would be surprised, whether my baby was dark or blond. Jon was sitting right beside me, with half of our gene pool, for all of them to see.

My first two days of this induction process were spent watching rented movies, reading, and playing Scrabble with Jon, amid my growing contractions. It was all in all fairly enjoyable, if you don't mind lying in bed all day, with an occasional tight squeeze in the stomach area. But on day three things changed: the drugs were kicking in. A maternity nurse looked at the register from the fetal monitor. "You're having some good contractions here, Lori," she said.

After my mother arrived from Colorado, where she had moved with her new husband, I felt somehow safer. After all, nothing bad can happen with your mother around, right?

"Hello, honey." She came right to my side and brushed my hair out of my face to give me a kiss. "How are you feeling?"

"Not that great right now."

"She feels terrible," Jon edited.

Sue and Joe had also visited, bringing a pizza. But I was forbidden to eat anything during induction. Sue entertained me with a new batch of hospital horror stories. A patient in the ER whose fever spiked had had some kind of "pearly substance" that Tim got out of his chest with a needle.

"Lovely," I said. Sue has a way of describing these things in elaborate, flowery detail. It had made me more nauseous than before.

While Sue and Joe were there, a huge crack of thunder ripped through the sky, sounding like a plane going through the sound barrier. Then it started to pour.

"We'd better get going," Joe said. "Call us when there's any news."

"Look, Lori." Sue gestured to the window.

There, as if framing the distant red rocks, were two bright, full horseshoes of color, bent over the sky. "Not just a single rainbow but a double," she said.

"It's good luck," I said, thinking of the fragmented rainbow I'd seen a few days before on my way back from Tuba City.

Rainbows are important in Navajo culture, woven into rug designs with rectangular faces at the bottoms, striped *yeis*, or Navajo gods. *Maybe it's a gift from Thomas,* I thought. *Maybe it's another prayer for me and Kodi.*

Afterward Dr. Waxman came by to take a look at me. After an excruciatingly painful bimanual exam, he placed an internal monitor into my uterus and ruptured the bag of amniotic fluid to speed up the labor process.

"Lori, I'll tell you," he said. "By now his head should be a lot lower down and engaged."

"And what does that mean?" I asked.

"Usually by thirty-six weeks that head is a lot lower down."

"Can you see that on the ultrasound?"

"Not always, but I can tell with my fingers. Right now your blood pressure looks good. The diastolic BP is down to where it's supposed to be. Let me check your reflexes."

"What's going to happen?"

He gave me the news. "This inches us a little closer to a C-section. But I'll tell you one thing, Lori. One way or another, by rounds tomorrow we'll have you and baby in postpartum."

"That's what I want to hear," I said.

Any woman who has ever had PIH knows the names of several substances: prostaglandin, a gel that dilates the cervix; pitosin, which helps the contractions; and lastly magnesium sulfate, an antiseizure drug that counteracts the preeclampsia or hypertension symptoms. Magnesium sulfate is by far the most obnoxious. By relaxing all the body's smooth muscles, it totally disables a person, rendering them a little stronger than a slab of Jell-O. It also has the charming quality of causing extreme nausea.

When they started me on magnesium sulfate, my life stretched out like slowly pulled taffy. I'd had a big dose, and it made me feel about ten degrees hotter than normal and a very weird combination of groggy, spacey, and just plain drained. My vision was blurred, and the light hurt my eyes so much, Jon put a warm washcloth over them. Even speaking became a strain. *I will have to remember this degree of misery when I am treating really sick patients,* I thought. *I will have to remember the way senses are altered.*

Since Jerry Choi, one of our best anesthesiologists, had put in my epidural, the contractions were now nothing, just a series of tightening sensations that grabbed my abdomen.

The nurse was checking the fetal monitor. Jerry adjusted some knobs for the epidural. Mom was sitting on one side of me, Jon on the other. *Get a few more people in here, and this could be like a traditional Navajo birth,* I thought, *with an entire community.*

As if reading my thoughts, there was a quick knock, and the door opened. In walked a middle-aged Navajo woman in street clothes, whom I had never seen before.

"Excuse me," she said. "I do not mean to intrude." My mother walked over to her and they went together into the hallway.

"I wonder what that was about," I said, peeking out from the washcloth.

Then the two women came back in. "Lori, this lady is Maria Herrera, a medicine woman related to one of the other women having a baby here tonight. She wants to know if you want her to do a prayer for the baby while she is here."

The woman smiled at me politely. It was all I could do to nod and smile weakly back.

Maria Herrera had brought a red sash, and she tied it in knots. She walked over to my side and placed it downward on my belly. Then she gestured to Jon. "Pull that out," she instructed him.

Jon did. Four times he pulled the knots out of the red sash over my belly. Then she placed the sash over me again and took out a leather medicine pouch, like Thomas's. From it she retrieved four little handfuls of corn pollen and sprinkled them on my belly in two stripes on either side of the sash. As she whispered a prayer I could hardly hear, I shut my eyes.

When I opened them, she was gone. "Tell me that really happened," I whispered to Jon. As soon as she left, I felt myself relax completely, and the sickening effect of the pitosin seemed to subside. I slept.

When I awakened someone else came in. What good spirit was entering this time? I wondered. It was Claire, on call for the night. She placed her hand gently on my belly. With her wire-rimmed glasses, short brown hair, and sensitivity, Claire was definitely cool.

"Is there anything I can do to make you more comfortable, Lori?" I shook my head with the two grams of energy left in my body. "Hopefully this will get things rolling. If it doesn't in a couple of hours, we'll consider this a failure."

"Okay," I said.

At ten o'clock Claire came back into the room. She did a quick pelvic exam and told me I was not dilating enough. "We're going to need to do a C-section soon," she said. "I'm sorry, Lori."

A state akin to sleep, but not sleep, came over me. It was sleep's mean little brother, who knocks you unconscious but makes sure you feel like hell anyway. When I awoke, Mom had her hand on my forehead. "Honey?" she said.

"I'm ready. Let's do it," I said.

Jerry Choi and several nurses helped me onto a gurney and wheeled me into the OR. I looked up to see Ella Mae Belinda, a Navajo nurse who had been in the OR with me hundreds of times. It was the strangest sensation to see her *above* me, as a patient would.

"Hi, Ella," I whispered. Claire, gowned and gloved, came into the OR. She and another scrub nurse screwed in the sterile light handles and draped me. Jerry had given me a zap of something strong because the world was going soft focus. From the corner of my eye, I recognized two other faces. One was Betty, a nurse friend, and the other was Sue. "Hi, Sue," I tried to say, but it came out a mumble.

"We're gonna start, Lori," Claire said.

It is the last thing I really remember. Sue later told me that Claire made a swift incision and placed the retractors in my lower abdomen with grace. "Perfect," Claire said. After cutting down through fascia and separating muscle, she said again, "That's perfect."

Then I remember blurred sounds, and a cry, a gurgly cry, and then the words, "Hi, sweetheart. You *are* handsome."

Jon whispered behind me, "He's blond!"

"He is not!" I tried to say.

Then Claire joked, "Lori, you want me to take out your gallbladder while I'm in here?"

I could not speak but felt like answering: "Sure, and bag it up for me, please!"

"Hand me the suture scissors, Anita," I heard her say. Then for a brief moment I saw a blurry purplish package, wrapped in a blanket. "Hi, Mom," a nurse said. "Say hi, baby."

▲▲▲▲

Kodi was born at seven pounds, four ounces. He flushed from purple to a soft pink color in minutes, and I sat mesmerized beside him for the rest of the night. We named him Christopher Kodiak Alvord, and he was honey colored, with dark hair (not blond!), and from the first moment I could see his Navajo ancestry, shining in his dark-lashed eyes.

For weeks, whenever I held Kodi to nurse or rocked him when he cried, I'd examine every detail of his face. He had a tiny crease on his chin and a plump lower lip that he sucked on when he was unhappy, and he tended to furrow his brow, as if he were a little worried. His face was one of the most amazing things I had ever looked at. For something so small, it seemed to have so many different expressions.

As I nursed him, fall came into the air with the smell of piñon smoke from all the fireplaces. One morning, when Jon went out to get some milk, a thin veil of ice had laced the truck windows. I still had not gone back to work, and we were exhausted from midnight feedings and the changing of Kodi's numerous tiny diapers, but it was still so exciting, each time we looked at him.

One day that autumn Jon and Kodi and I drove to the top of Mount Taylor. There we dug a small but deep hole, too deep for the coyotes to smell, and covered his placenta and umbilical cord with cold, soft earth. Sacred Mount Taylor was where I chose to bury it, so that Kodi would always remember who he was, honor the people he was descended from, and always respect their ways.

I could now speak from personal experience about the combination of Western medicine and Navajo ways: It had produced my beautiful, healthy baby boy.

There was only one thing we were waiting for—to hear Christopher Kodiak Alvord laugh.

Chapter Fourteen

▲▲▲▲

MOUNT TAYLOR IN THE
REARVIEW MIRROR

*Yesterday, turning south for New Mexico at
San Luis, Coyote looked at the mountains
and said, "We'll see you again." And prayed
for safety, strength, and the ability to see
beauty.*

—SIMON ORTIZ[9]

I n B.J.'s bedroom in Mescalero, New Mexico,
Grandma lay still in a few scattered rays of light on
the cot that had been unfolded for her. When I
walked in and saw her lying there, I was puzzled.
She seemed different somehow, surrounded by a
circle of neatly placed brown drink coasters.

The day before, Jon had gone on a ski trip. I had
driven down to Mescalero with Grandma and
Kodi, who was almost two, to meet my mother and
visit my little sister Robyn. It was a celebratory
visit. Robyn and her boyfriend, Verlyn, had married
the year before, and she had recently given birth to
their first daughter, Annika. We'd gotten in late the
night before, and after admiring the dark-eyed
newborn with her soft tuft of chestnut hair, we had
all gone right to bed.

In the morning we were having coffee, when I realized Grandma hadn't gotten up yet. I went to check on her. She was lying in the exact position I'd seen her in the night before, on her back, with one arm drawn up over her eyes.

"Grandma," I said, gently touching her arm to awaken her. She was warm but did not respond. "Grandma!" I repeated. Kodi and B.J. were behind me, peeking in the door. I uncovered her face and touched her chin. When I opened her eyes to see her pupils, I knew.

We called the ambulance but feared the worst. As Verlyn and I guessed, she had had a massive stroke—her brain had hemorrhaged. The doctor gave her about twenty-four hours to remain alive.

The night before, she had played a game with two-year-old Kodi. He would hand her a coaster, and she would hand it back. Over and over they played this game. Kodi laughed and laughed—he had never seemed to tire of it, nor had she. Earlier that morning I saw him wander into her room carrying the stack of coasters. It must have been he who had laid them out like that around her, trying to stir her into playing with him again.

Amazingly, my *shínálí* Grace lived another week, but she never woke up again. It was long enough, however, for her to be brought home to Gallup, some seven and a half hours away. Not until she was at GIMC and some of her relatives, her sister Janice and her cousins, visited her, did she let go of this world. Although she had no birth certificate, her relatives estimated her age to be about ninety-one years.

It was incredible to me, the graceful and peaceful way she left us. She had seen her newest great-grandchild. Then she had waited, semiconscious in a coma, to die in Dinetah, surrounded by her sacred mountains, where she could feel at home. In so many ways, it was the way she should go. For some time her mind had wandered, and she'd been forgetful.

We'd feared it was the onset of dementia or Alzheimer's. She would not have wanted to live like that.

But more amazing still was the timing. I had asked Jon on the phone: "Did you tell her?"

"I didn't," he said. "I didn't want her to worry about it."

"Neither did I," I said.

"She must have guessed."

We were talking about the job offer I had received. I'd been asked to move back to New Hampshire to work at Dartmouth Medical School.

"Grandma was so intuitive," I said. "She must have somehow known and decided—there was no way on earth she was moving to New Hampshire!" She had always been strong-willed, and full of self-determination. She had simply decided it was time to go, and once we brought her home, she did it her way. I had heard stories about how older Navajos were able to choose their time of death. I'd always thought that was something that happened long ago, but now I wondered. My biggest reservation about moving to New Hampshire had been how Grandma would handle all the ice and snow, and being away from *Dinétah*.

The idea of moving had been a surprise, even to me. I was happy in Gallup, I loved my practice and my patients and the surgical group I worked with. I had not looked for another job. Like everything else in my life—my decision to attend Dartmouth as an undergraduate, my last-minute decision to apply to medical school, my eleventh-hour choice to become a surgeon, even my choice of a husband—this next turn in life was to be abrupt and completely unforeseen. But as a longtime believer that a higher power operated my life as if it were a roadster, moving me on and off life's ramps and exits before I had time to blink, I was growing fairly used to the unexpected.

The job had come about through Gordon Russell, a Dartmouth alumnus, chairman of the board of overseers for Dartmouth Medical School, and a longtime friend and advocate of the Native American Program at Dartmouth. One day, out of the blue, he called me and mentioned that the medical school had a position open for associate dean of student affairs. He asked if I would be interested in applying for it. I swallowed hard. "I would certainly consider it," I said.

I went home and thought about it. Was this the right step for me? Was I the right person for them?

Like a book that could be read only a few pages at a time, my understanding of how Navajo philosophy could help me practice medicine was gradually evolving and expanding, and I had really been focused on this inner journey. Walking in Beauty had already taught me so much and helped me "unlearn" many concepts I had been taught in my medical training.

I had learned how to respect my patients and empower them. I had learned how important it is to acknowledge and value each member of the medical team. I had learned that when it comes to treating patients' illness, everything matters: our efforts, their efforts, their spiritual health, the health of their relationships, their comfort with and trust in the procedure they would undergo.

I had been hesitant to share these "discoveries" with others, particularly surgeons, because they were so different from the usual attitudes toward surgical practice, and because I had not yet had a clear understanding of their depth and breadth.

In addition, articulating these thoughts was not always easy, and I wasn't sure people wanted to hear them anyway. If it was important for other people to learn these things, I thought, then they would learn about them in their own ways. In typical Navajo fashion, I did little to promote them. But the outside world *was* often interested, and in atypical Navajo fashion, I did not turn it away.

I had often been asked to speak at commencement ceremonies at Navajo high schools and at universities like the University of Northern Colorado, Northern Arizona University,

Bates College, and Stanford Medical School. Articles about my work and philosophy had followed, in the *Chicago Tribune* and *The New York Times*. They were then syndicated and published all over the country. Word was leaking out, slowly, about these ideas. I was asked to speak to conference planners for the National Institutes of Health Office of Research on Women's Health at a symposium titled Research on Women's Health for the Twenty-first Century.

In general the audiences were very enthusiastic. Clearly, people at the end of our century were searching for a different, better, and more sensitive kind of medicine. Still, what would the people at an esteemed college like Dartmouth think about these concepts?

I soon had a chance to find out. After I sent in my application and had a few initial telephone conversations, I received an invitation to come to New Hampshire for an interview. During two days' worth of interviews, I talked about my evolving sense of the need for medicine to make some vital changes. As I spoke, the people who were listening seemed to understand my passion and dedication.

"Navajo people," I told them, "have a concept called *"Hózhóné háaz'dlíí,"* Walking in Beauty, but it isn't the beauty that most people think of. Beauty to Navajos means living in balance and harmony with yourself and the world. It means caring for yourself—mind, body, and spirit—and having the right relationships with your family, community, the animal world, the environment—earth, air, and water—our planet and universe.

"If a person respects and honors all these relationships," I said, "then they will be Walking in Beauty."

In the Western world, I explained, disease is very compartmentalized by organs or medical specialties, and in some ways this does not benefit the patient. Specialists often don't look outside their own parameters to see what else might be influencing an illness.

A Navajo healer, I explained, will look at the person's

whole life and the lives of those around him or her. Usually, the healer has lived in the same community with the person for decades; he knows a great deal about the person and what might be happening in his or her life. The Navajo view is a macro view, whereas Western medicine often takes a micro view.

A person might be sick because he treats his wife, children, or elders unkindly, or has a bad attitude toward his neighbors, or has neglected his body and become lazy and fat. He may be too absorbed in acquiring wealth or other personal gains and has neglected those around him. A Navajo healer will look for the imbalance. To a *hataałii* it is clear that everything affects everything else. The stress from disharmony can cause physical sickness, depression, even violence and death.

If the concept of balance is extended to the community level, then communities out of balance will have problems such as gang violence, elder neglect, child abuse, and drug use. As Western society has moved to a focus on the individual rather than the community, the support and sanctions of the community have faded away. In traditional Native societies, youth have great respect for elders for their wisdom, there is no such thing as orphanages, and children are cared for and valued by the entire community. Apply this same concept to the national level, and it is clear that if nations do not live in harmony together, then wars are a natural result. Now in the nuclear age, the health of all humanity weighs in the balance.

An imbalance of humans with the natural world also leads to illness. While it may not seem obvious, an imbalance in the natural world can have disastrous consequences. Native people have always been careful to respect the animal world. Many tribes feel that humans are not superior to animals and that animals have spirits as well.

Living in balance with the rest of the animal world has protected species for millennia—but Western society does not share the view that this is essential. Now many species are being sacrificed and exterminated by humans, either deliberately or as a result of carelessness. It is hard for Native people to believe that humans could be so uncaring as to wipe another species off the face of the earth, but it is happening all around us now. And it is not only the animal world that is under attack, but the environment as well.

In time, since we live in a closely interrelated ecosystem, one of these careless acts could backfire and put the human species itself at risk for extinction. Human health is dependent upon planetary health. All must exist in a delicate web of balanced relationships.

In the Navajo world the sun, water, weather, forests, and other living creatures are all considered to have spirit and life. They are considered family, and even called "Mother Earth, Father Sky," and animals are "brother" and "sister." This reverence for our planet has protected it for thousands of years, but now it lies in grave jeopardy.

Walking in Beauty, a broad approach to health, illness, and life, I explained, had become the cornerstone of my philosophy, relevant to me in both my personal life and my surgical practice. As I attempted to create harmonious relationships within my personal life and within the staff at GIMC, life had become less stressful and more meaningful.

I began to understand the importance of establishing the right relationships with my patients. This interaction was a spiritual relationship, just as medicine men see their relationships to their patients. I wanted to teach medical students to set out to treat each patient encounter as having a sacred component, in which the patient's mental-spiritual health required as much attention as their body.

I needed the patients' spirits to assist me in surgery, and their minds should be relaxed and in a state of trust before they went to the operating room. They should be prepared to let me enter the sacred chambers of their bodies. Their spirits and mine had to work together to allow the process of healing to occur.

While I did not always come right out and say it to every patient, I worked hard to bring them to the point of trust and a place where they could accept the operation and view themselves as my partner, participating in their healing and getting well.

Bringing the patients' spirits into the healing process was having results: I was seeing many fewer complications, and the patients were happier.

I also told my interviewers about what I thought would be a perfect hospital. It would be a place where patients felt cared for, listened to, and integral to their treatment. Because for Navajos, harmony, beauty, and wellness are intertwined, it would be housed in a physically beautiful building. Most importantly, those who practiced there would be healers as well as doctors.

The ideal hospital would not smell like a hospital; nor would it necessarily look like a hospital. Perhaps it would have adobe walls and fresh, clean, natural smells. It would be light filled and warm, with generous and comfortable seating for relatives. The windows would not be square and chrome but rather round or arched. There would be porches, flowers, and gardens. In addition to state-of-the art operating rooms and equipment, there would be a ceremonial space, for use by any who felt the need for it. People who speak the language of the patients would be there at all times.

When patients entered—whether to have chemotherapy, a surgical procedure, or a baby—they would feel that every person they encountered, be it an X-ray technician, a nurse, a receptionist, or a surgeon, was committed to their comfort and was participating in their healing process. It would be a place where illness was thought of not as a matter of a single organ or bodily system but rather as the effect of an imbalance. It

would see illness as a lack of harmony in any part of a patient's world: their physical body, their mind, their spirit, their
relations with family and friends, their community, their nation, or their environment. Nations at war, toxic pollutants in
the environment, and depletion of natural resources all threaten
our existence on the planet and affect health—mental, physical, and spiritual. The doctors in my hospital would recognize this. They would think of helping their patients in terms
of restoring balance to their lives. Instead of the compartmentalized specialties, doctors would share discoveries that
would have beneficial effects in other areas of their patients'
lives.

My ideal operating room would have a team of people who
worked together smoothly and easily, with respect for one another and their patients. Each member, no matter what their
rank, would be considered important and invaluable. I had
formed this daydream during my years working with Lujan
and at GIMC, caring for Native patients. But I felt deeply
that the ramifications could be great for the larger medical
system.

My thoughts were well received by the leaders at Dartmouth
Medical School—there was an openness to new ideas that I
liked—and I left with a good feeling about the encounter.

Meanwhile, even as I was imagining this perfect hospital, others were thinking in a similar fashion. People everywhere, from all walks of life—other physicians, health care
providers, and people at large in society—were calling for
change in the health care system. Wherever I lectured, people would come up to me afterward and tell me stories of
their impersonal treatment by doctors, of problems getting
appropriate treatment through managed care programs, and
of doctors or hospital staff who had treated them insensi-
tively. They felt powerless, often miserable inside hospitals,
stripped of their dignity.

Nurses would tell me that they felt disrespected by doctors. Physicians would tell me that they wanted doctoring to

go back to the old ways, when they were known and trusted by their communities and families. "That kind of practice is hard to find," they'd say, "but it is more fulfilling."

They complained of health care systems that require them to see a new patient every fifteen minutes. "How can we build relationships when we are forced to spend so little time with them?" they asked.

I do not know the answer. But what works for me, whether I have five or fifty-five minutes, is to give myself completely to my patient for that time. I listen carefully to them and let them know that my attention is completely focused on them and that this is their time. It isn't the entire answer, but it helps.

Meanwhile a new breed of clinical studies have been released further supporting my beliefs. They show that patients fare better when they feel a sense of community. Breast cancer patients fare better when they are in support groups; even people who have pets fare better. Respected journals like *The American Journal of Epidemiology* report that social activities and relationships are "inversely related to mortality rates." In the same journal a study reported that social factors, including "religious commitment, the proximity and number of living offspring," cause lower mortality in the elderly. A report in *The Journal of the American Medical Association* revealed that the National Institutes of Health has funded a study of the feelings of spirituality of patients and their effects on mental and physical health.

The studies confirm everything I have been learning—and show the multifactorial nature of illness and healing, the importance of maintaining healthy relationships in every part of one's life, and that healers should take into account that whole life. Attitudes were changing in the larger world of health care, beginning to mirror my own. The time has come for a critical shift in the practice and delivery of medicine. It is ironic that so-called "primitive cultures" such as the Navajo have understood these concepts for hundreds, perhaps thousands, of years.

After another visit to Dartmouth and a round of interviews with the surgical staff, the job offer came. Andy Wallace, dean of Dartmouth Medical School, called to offer me the position of associate dean of student affairs.

Part of me was not surprised—I had seen the trajectory of my life curving nine months earlier, after speaking with Gordon Russell. But another part of me was completely stunned, the part of me that still saw herself as a Navajo girl playing on a mesa in a remote corner of New Mexico.

It had been hard enough to reconcile my simple past and my culture with my surgical training, and although I had considered doing additional projects, I would never have predicted this. I thought about the downsides: I would have to leave my people and leave my spiritual home, the beautiful Southwest. I would leave good friends behind.

Some of my Navajo friends and family were concerned: "Will you be all right?" they kept asking. "How long must you stay away?"

It would be a major sacrifice for me to be away from my tribe. I didn't know how long I would be able to stay in New Hampshire. I had worked hard to build a practice that was sensitive to the needs of Navajo patients, and now my tribal home *did* feel like putting on soft, comfortable moccasins.

Then I thought of the benefits. For Navajo people, I would be breaking another glass ceiling, which might make it easier for others to follow a medical path in the future. Navajo people take pride in any advancement that any member makes. It helps prove that Navajo people can do anything that anyone from any other culture can do (and sometimes better). This encouragement and confidence building was something I had spent many hours talking to young people about. I wanted Navajo people to believe in themselves and to be strong.

On another level, I hoped I could learn more about managing health care systems, since Navajo people would soon be operating their own health care system, independent of the IHS, and I hoped to assist in this transition, or be of use to my tribe at some point in the future.

One of my own long-term goals was to gain the ability to help improve national health care policies for Native Americans. I would have greater opportunity to do this if I accepted the position. I would have the opportunity to teach the principles of Walking in Beauty, the ultimate medicine gift. Going to New Hampshire was a chance to give back all I'd learned.

In fact, no decision had to be made—this was what I was supposed to do, and I recognized this as the next part of my "life trail." Jon was very excited. Having grown up in Utah, he loved snow and winter sports and was completely supportive of the move.

We found a Cape-style house on a hill overlooking Lake Mascoma, surrounded by birds and trees. From there, importantly, we had a long-range view of the horizon. I wouldn't feel claustrophobic. The natural beauty was nourishing and inspiring.

The whole planet is inside the four sacred mountains if you think about it, I joked to myself, *since the planet is round.*

We met the moving van with the rest of our lives, and a few days later I began my new job. I would work as a general surgeon 40 percent of the time at Dartmouth Medical Center, and at the medical school 60 percent of the time.

At the Dartmouth-Hitchcock Medical Center I noticed some interesting things. The hospital is modern and painted white with green trim. It is surrounded by an idyllic forest, with tall pine maple, and birch trees all around. In the center is a glass atrium rotunda, flooded with sunlight, and the roofs of the main walkway open to huge skylights. Along the main floor a cluster of shops and restaurants beckons—including a small dry cleaner and a bank. How convenient for patients and staff, I thought. A glass-enclosed restaurant looks out on the surrounding timberland. It was the most beautiful hospital I had ever seen.

Then I noticed other, subtler things. It didn't smell like a hospital. The light was often natural, and there were no intercom pages. The atmosphere was one of cheerfulness, spaciousness, and serenity. People were working to make this hospital a "healing environment," where patients felt comfortable and where the natural environment—the trees, sun, and sky—were invited to come as close as possible, to encourage healing as well.

Some parts of the hospital seemed to be moving rapidly toward the ideal. The Children's Hospital at Dartmouth and the birthing pavilion resembled an interior decorator's showroom for "casual living," complete with toys and an aquarium for children and Jacuzzis for women in labor.

One day I was astonished to find a flyer posted for a conference on spirituality and medicine. The conference had several sessions, one of which dealt with "the art of using patient's beliefs to improve clinical outcome." I knew then that the importance of harmony, of *hózhǫ́*, was starting to be recognized in the Dartmouth medical community.

The hospital didn't have adobe walls, and roasted green chili is virtually unknown in New England. But it was very much like my dream hospital.

▲▲▲▲

The first time I was in Hanover, years ago, I was sixteen years old and felt invisible; I had not known what I wanted to do with my life or what I was capable of. My life was the meeting place for two worlds in constant collision. Like most other Dartmouth alums, I still carried deep, intense feelings for this college. I was pleased to find that the atmosphere for Native Americans and women was much more inviting; the student body was far more diverse than it had been when I was a student. I never dreamed I would return as a member of the Medical School faculty and administration.

Sometimes the demands I now have seem overwhelming: the directors of the offices of student affairs, minority affairs, financial aid, the registrar, admissions, and the advising dean all report to me.

I work with the four other associate deans to assist the dean of the Medical School and help with the long-term planning for the school, in everything from budgetary and curriculum issues to new program development. The work is challenging and exciting because I am learning so many new things.

I was delighted to find that Dartmouth offers a rotation to medical schools at Tuba City, Arizona, another IHS hospital that offers care to Navajo and Hopi patients. This rotation could definitely help students understand Navajo thinking about medicine. Students also rotate to Bethel, Alaska, to work with the IHS doctors there.

In my other office, at the hospital, I prepare for surgery and check up on surgical cases through a sophisticated computer program for tracking patients, which I can use to review patients' progress with "electronic charts."

But most importantly, I now have the opportunity to teach Dartmouth medical students how to respect their privilege of placing their hands inside another human being. I have a chance to explain the importance of gaining patient trust, of giving back power to patients, of relieving their fear and anxiety—and the impact this has on healing. In my initial address to the incoming first- and second-year med school classes, I spoke of all these things that have become essential to me, and of how I first learned them by returning to my tribe's ancient beliefs.

Afterward a woman from the class came up to me. She waited patiently for others to ask questions, then asked me shyly, "Dr. Alvord, I liked so much what you said about Navajo beliefs, but I am wondering—do these concepts have relevance for other cultures, for non-Indian peoples?"

It was the question I had been asking myself for years, and I finally felt safe giving the answer I had come to believe: "Absolutely," I said. "They absolutely do."

There is a story Navajo people tell their children about how *Hosteen* Owl and *Hosteen* Bat brought medicine to the Fire People. *Hosteen* Owl helps tie a medicine bundle on Bat's back. " *'This is all little Bat will need to accomplish his mission,'* said *Hosteen* Owl, *'. . . and this is all the . . . herb medicine I brought from the lower world. It contains much magic and I have given it for the benefit of all the people living in the new land.' "*[10]

The last day I was in Gallup, I thought of the story, and my heart felt lighter. I felt I was doing the right thing in this dramatic move back East.

Maybe like Owl and Bat, who brought medicine to the people, I could help share Navajo ideas about healing with the rest of the world, to help change the course of medicine. This medicine has its own path and journey; my role is simply to help facilitate this leg of it.

Things are changing in other places, too. At the request of the All Indian Pueblo Council, Lujan accepted their nomination to be a trustee of the University of New Mexico Hospital. I was pleased at the news. *This will be another way that the concerns of Native people will be heard,* I thought.

On our last day in New Mexico, as we drove from Gallup to Albuquerque to catch the plane to New Hampshire, we passed the beautiful red sandstone mesas and bluffs that stretch along I-40, and we passed mile marker 47.

I won't be gone long, I whispered to my father. As we continued eastward, I glanced up and saw Mount Taylor's snow-capped peak shining in the rearview mirror. I thought of Kodi's placenta, buried on the highest peak. My eyes clouded with tears.

I am taking you with me, I thought, *if only in my heart.*

NOTES

1. Aileen O'Bryan, *Navajo Indian Myths* (New York: Dover, 1994).

2. Raymond Friday Locke, *The Book of the Navajo,* fifth edition (Mankind Publishing Co., 1992).

3. Aileen O'Bryan, Ibid.

4. Ibid.

5. Simon J. Ortiz, *Going for the Rain: Poems* (New York: Harper and Row, 1976).

6. Stephen Kunitz and Jerrold Levy, *Drinking Careers: A Twenty-Five-Year Study of Three Navajo Populations* (New Haven: Yale University Press, 1994), p. 1.

7. George W. Cronyn, ed., *American Indian Poetry* (New York: Ballantine, 1962).

8. Monty Roessel, "The Long Walk: Retracing the Navajo's Trail of Tears," *New Mexico* (August 1993), p. 74.

9. Simon J. Ortiz, Ibid.

10. Frank Newcomb, *Navajo Folk Tales* (Albuquerque: University of New Mexico Press, 1967).

GLOSSARY
OF NAVAJO TERMS

Ahéhee' thank you

'Ashchí to give birth

Ashįįhi Dineé the salt people clan, one of the original clans of the Navajo tribe

'Ałkidáá' many years ago

'Ałní a person who is a "half breed" or has two different heritages

'Ats'íís naałzid cancer; literally "a body that is rotting"

Ayóó ninshné I love you

Azee Al'i Hotsaai' hospital; literally, "the big space where medicine is given"

Azee'iiłini na'atgizhii surgeon

Bilagáana Anglo; white person

Blessing Way a traditional healing ceremony

Ch'įįndi the ghost of a dead person that comes back to inflict pain or suffering on the living

Dibé Ntsaa the northern sacred mountain

Diné the Navajo people; literally, "the people"

Dinétah the place of the Navajo people

Dook'o'oosłííd the western sacred mountain

Dootl'izhii At'eed Turquoise Girl, a character in traditional Navajo folklore; one of the first women

Haashch'ééłtíí Talking God

Hataałii medicine person; medicine man; literally "singer"

Hogan traditional Navajo eight-sided dwelling structure, whose door faces east

Hosteen Mr.; an address of respect

Hózhǫ́ or *hózhǫ́ni* beauty, harmony (a concept of living in harmony and balance)

Hózhǫ́ne háaz'dlíí "it is beautiful all around me"

Kinaałdá Navajo four-day ceremony that is given for girls when they become women (at puberty)

Kiva a round room that is wholly or partially underground, used ceremonially by Pueblo tribes and Anasazi (the "ancient ones") cliff dwellers

ł a sound close to "lth"

Na'agizh surgery; literally "to cut open"

Naasht'e'zhí Zuni (one of the pueblo tribes in New Mexico)

Nádziih to heal, to clear up

Natzee cancer, "something that rots"

Night Chant a traditional nine-night healing ceremony, held in the winter. Sand paintings are made and other blessings performed, including dancing, prayers, and the use of corn pollen placed on various parts of the sick person's body

Shalako a traditional ceremony held annually in December by the Zuni people, to bless their new houses

Shimasání maternal grandmother

Shínálí paternal grandmother

Shush bear

Sisna'jin the eastern sacred mountain

Skinwalker a spirit of a dead or living person who can change into the shape of an animal, most often a wolf

Tse yik'áán Hogback Mountains

Tsi'naajinii A Navajo clan, literally "the black-streaked wood people," who came from a forest of trees with black bark; one of the bear group of clans

Tsoodził Mount Taylor, the southern sacred mountain

Wedding Basket Ceremony traditional Navajo marriage ceremony, in which a basket of corn pollen paste is passed around to a group of relatives and everyone must take a pinch and eat it.

Yáat'ééh hello, greetings

Yeibechei a ceremony held on the last night of a Night Chant, in which all the Gods, including Talking God, come to visit the sick person

Yikáísdah the Milky Way

Zuni an ancient southwestern Indian tribe that neighbors the Navajo nation. According to their beliefs, they are the descendants of the ancient cliff-dwelling peoples known as the Anasazi.

▲▲▲▲

BIBLIOGRAPHY

Bulow, Ernie. *Navajo Taboos*. Gallup, NM: Buffalo Medicine Books, 1991.

Cronyn, George W., ed. *American Indian Poetry*. New York: Ballantine, 1962.

Dutton, Bertha P. *American Indians of the Southwest*. Albuquerque: University of New Mexico Press, 1974.

Garrod, Andrew, et al., eds. *First Person, First Peoples: Native American College Graduates Tell Their Stories*. Ithaca, NY: Cornell University Press, 1997.

Kunitz, Stephen, and Jerrold Levy. *Drinking Careers: A Twenty-Five-Year Study of Three Navajo Populations*. New Haven: Yale University Press, 1994.

Locke, Raymond Friday. *The Book of the Navajo*. 5th ed. Los Angeles: Mankind Publishing Company, 1992.

O'Bryan, Aileen. *Navajo Indian Myths*. New York: Dover, 1994.

Ortiz, Simon. *Going for the Rain*. New York: Harper and Row, 1976.

Roessel, Monty. "The Long Walk: Retracing the Navajo's Trail of Tears." *New Mexico,* August 1993.

Russell, Sharman Apt. *Songs of the Flute Player: Seasons in the Life of the Southwest.* Reading, MA: Addison Wesley, 1991.

Weatherford, Jack. *Indian Givers: How the Indians of the Americas Transformed the World.* New York: Fawcett Columbine, 1988.

Young, Robert W., and William Morgan. *Colloquial Navajo, A Dictionary.* New York: Hippocrene Books, 1994.

▲▲▲▲

ABOUT THE AUTHORS

LORI ARVISO ALVORD, M.D., is the recipient of the New Mexico Governor's Award for Outstanding Women and has been awarded a Certificate of Appreciation from the Eastern Navajo Health Board for her service to the Navajo people. Currently "on sabbatical" from the Navajo Nation, Lori is serving on the faculty of Dartmouth Medical School, in Hanover, New Hampshire, as associate dean of student affairs (and minority affairs) and assistant professor of surgery. Lori and her husband, Jonathan, have two children—Kodiak and Kaitlyn—and live in New Hampshire.

ELIZABETH COHEN VAN PELT has written for *The New York Times*, the *New York Post*, *People*, *Glamour*, *Rolling Stone*, *Family Circle*, and many other publications. She currently lives in Colesville, New York, where she is a reporter for the *Press & Sun-Bulletin* [Binghamton] and in New York City with her husband, Shane Van Pelt, and their daughter, Ava.

To download a study guide for *The Scalpel and the Silver Bear*, visit www.bantamdell.com.